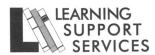

FORTHCOMING TITLES

Occupational Therapy for the Brain-Injured Adult
Jo Clark-Wilson and Gordon Muir Giles

Physiotherapy in Respiratory Care
A problem-solving approach
Alexandra Hough

Speech and Language Problems in Children
Dilys A. Treharne

THERAPY IN PRACTICE SERIES
Edited by Jo Campling

This series of books is aimed at 'therapists' concerned with rehabilitation in a very broad sense. The intended audience particularly includes occupational therapists, physiotherapists and speech therapists, but many titles will also be of interest to nurses, psychologists, medical staff, social workers, teachers or volunteer workers. Some volumes are interdsiciplinary, others are aimed at one particular profession. All titles will be comprehensive but concise, and practical but with due reference to relevant theory and evidence. They are not research monographs but focus on professional practice, and will be of value to both students and qualified personnel.

Breakdown of Speech

Causes and remediation

NANCY R. MILLOY, Ph.D, M.Sc., Dip.CST, MCST,

CHAPMAN AND HALL
LONDON • NEW YORK • TOKYO • MELBOURNE • MADRAS

UK   Chapman and Hall, 2–6 Boundary Row, London SE1 8HN

USA   Chapman and Hall, 29 West 35th Street, New York NY10001

JAPAN   Chapman and Hall Japan, Thomson Publishing Japan, Hirakawacho Nemoto Building, 7F, 1–7–11 Hirakawa-cho, Chiyoda-ku, Tokyo 102

AUSTRALIA Chapman and Hall Australia, Thomas Nelson Australia, 102 Dodds Street, South Melbourne, Victoria 3205

INDIA   Chapman and Hall India, R. Seshadri, 32 Second Main Road, CIT East, Madras 600 035

First edition 1991

© 1991 Nancy R. Milloy

Phototypeset in 10/12pt Times by Input Typesetting, London
Printed in Great Britain by St Edmundsbury Press Ltd,
Bury St Edmunds, Suffolk

ISBN 0 412 31550 5

British Library Cataloguing in Publication Data
Milloy, Nancy R.
   Breakdown of Speech.
   1. Man. Language disorders & speech
   I. Title   II. Series
   616.855

   ISBN 0–412–31550–5

Library of Congress Cataloging-in-Publication Data
Milloy, Nancy R., 1927–
   Breakdown of Speech: causes and remediation / Nancy R. Milloy.
       p.   cm. – (Therapy in practice)
   Includes bibliographical references (p.   ) and indexes.
   ISBN 0–412–31550–5
   1. Speech disorders.   2. Speech – Physiological aspects.   3. Speech therapy.
   I. Title.   II. Series.
   RC423.M5554 1991
   616.85'5 – dc20   90–2058
                                            CIP

To Alex and Jean

Contents

Acknowledgements

I wish to thank the following people for their support in the preparation of this book: Jane Russell, Sheila Hardy and Rae Smith who contributed in their different areas of expertise; my colleagues and friends who patiently listened and advised, and particularly my husband, without whose help and encouragement it would have been difficult to complete the work.

Introduction

Be a craftsman in speech, so that thou mayest be strong, for the tongue is a sword, and speech is more valorous than any fighting.

Egyptian Proverb

The first duty of a man is to speak; that is his chief business in this world.

R. L. Stevenson
Memories and Portraits, 1888

Communication is of paramount importance to people. After the 1939–45 war Winston Churchill changed from his fighting attitude and advised world planners to adopt 'jaw, nor war'. The present 'glasnost' is also reliant on the power of speech which, when used at its highest level, facilitates understanding. Only human beings possess this power.

To illustrate how the acceptance of the automatic nature of speech has come about, consider the following clinical examples.

Michael, aged 5;0, is one of identical twins. They have an elder brother of 8;0. Michael has severe cerebral palsy. His brothers are both normal healthy boys. Despite their mother's experience with his brothers, her greatest hope for Michael was to see him walking. However, after recent discussion and consideration of the situation she is now determined to help Michael to learn to communicate by whatever means is available to him. She has realized that the essence of a person is in being able to express feelings, desires and opinions as well as in being mobile.

Similarly, Julie's parents realized in time that early surgical intervention is critical to enable her to produce clear, non-nasal speech rather than to make her cosmetic appearance their first consideration. Julie was born with a unilateral cleft in her lip and palate. As she develops, plastic surgery will be used to realign her nose and lip to make them as near to normal as possible. Society still finds it difficult not to judge by appearances.

The aims of this book are to increase awareness of speech development and skills and to explore some means by which improvements may be achieved when those skills are absent or disrupted. The contents include current thinking from research and recent literature, management techniques particularly designed for students and newly qualified therapists, and comments considered helpful to parents, teachers and carers.

Hearing loss and deafness and their consequent effects on the development of speech have been dealt with in depth in other places. The result of the presence of one or other of these disabilities is here regarded as a language disorder and not a speech disorder. Reference is made to the learned articulation disorder which occasionally accompanies hearing loss.

Where direct quotes are made the authors' original text is adhered to strictly.

Each chapter stands alone. Chapter 1 discusses the production of speech and how it works. Language and speech are defined in the context of the subject-matter to be covered. Modifications to fundamental human processes and systems required to facilitate the production of spoken language are dealt with and discussed in terms of current research.

Chapter 2 highlights the relevant genetic and structural deviations from normal development which may lead to the production of disordered speech. Management of children with such deviations is considered and techniques of approach discussed.

The third and fourth chapters concentrate on what can go wrong with human neuromusculature and motor planning to prevent the acquisition of intelligible speech. The discussion ranges across the whole spectrum from laying down motor memories to carrying out reliable, automatic motor movements. Maturational development is also considered. Environmental factors such as parental influence, home background, sibling and other familial relationships are included for consideration. Basic interactional states between the child and those around him/her, particularly his/her parents, receive attention. Specific reference is made in Chapter 5 to types of disorders of fluency in children and current therapies are reviewed.

Voice disorders in children are covered in the sixth chapter and clinical management is detailed, for this and all other disorders dealt with.

Adolescent and adult speech difficulties comprise the remainder of this book, in Chapters 7 to 9. They have been treated in a slightly different manner. Chapter 7 includes the whole gamut of speech disorders found in the mature population ranging from teenage through young adulthood, middle age, to the elderly and extreme old age. The maintenance and repair of all forms of speech disorder is dealt with in Chapters 8 and 9.

The impossibility of divorcing speech and language has been acknowledged throughout the course of this book and inevitable references to language are made as required. Speech/language disorders are seen as learning disorders and aspects of this fact are included in several of the discussions which arise.

This book is aimed primarily at helping speech therapists and speech therapy students to direct their attention to the non-linguistic aspects of speech and particularly to emphasize the need for the physical 'readiness' which is necessary to precede the acquisition and development of language. The importance of counselling parents, teachers, play-group leaders and others instrumental in guiding the development of speech also features in the compilation of this work.

Emphasis is put on the fact that intervention in most types of speech and language disorder will usually be somewhat time-consuming. Many factors contribute to most cases and formed habits often have to be broken as well as new techniques learned in the course of improving production of speech. Account of the additional factor of maturation with children must always be taken. In severe cases, intervention becomes as necessary as other forms of learning and should be part of daily living. Where the problem is less severe, trends indicate that speech therapists frequently plan short, intensive treatment approaches accompanied and followed by support from parents, teachers and others. Reviews and 'topping-up' sessions are then arranged.

1

Speech versus language

As recently as 40 years ago there was no real appreciation of the dichotomy between speech and language. The speech therapy profession in the UK was founded at a time when the comprehension of human communication was based on the tangible aspects of speech.

These were seen as being almost entirely functional and mechanical with little or no reference to the cognitive and philosophical aspects of the subject. In the 1950s, descriptive linguists began to attempt to account for the forms and components of language and emphasis shifted to studying the grammar of language, thus concentrating on its structure (Bloomfield, 1933; Miller, 1951; Chomsky, 1957). Numerous studies followed and it would have been possible at that time to believe that human language was confined to its structure, such as subject, verb and object ordering, because so much emphasis was put on this area. It was only later that researchers started to investigate the possibilities of meaningfulness as an aspect of language, and even more recently that interest has been directed to the actual use made of language by human beings. This has led to the present consuming interest in pragmatics and discourse (Halliday, 1975; Bates, 1976; Kempson, 1977; Tough, 1977; Prutting, 1982; Wardough, 1985; Beveridge and Conti-Ramsden, 1987; Smith, 1988). These and other language studies and clinical discussions have effectively started to explain and clarify most aspects of the content, form and use of English (Bloom and Lahey, 1978). For example, language can be divided into the following components:

1. semantics   – pertaining to meaning and meaningfulness;
2. syntax   – pertaining to the order and structure of sentences;

3. morphology – pertaining to the structure of words;
4. phonology   – pertaining to the abstract linguistic level of individuals' sound systems;
5. pragmatics – pertaining to individuals' choice of words, use of language in social interaction and the effects of its use.

However, as a result of the direction that recent investigations have taken, the physical and mechanical aspects of language production have been neglected. Human language is only possible when the two aspects interact. The aim of this book is to concentrate on the physical modality of language.

WORKING DEFINITIONS

It may be useful to attempt to define language and speech. The former defies a simple definition as it is manifested by so many variables. However, a working definition for the purpose of this discussion could be as follows:

Language is a communication code consisting of the use of selected signals, signs and symbols to represent each aspect of that code and determined by cognitive rules dependent on learned cerebral function.

The definition of speech then could be:

Speech is an aspect of language represented by the use of signals produced by means of human exhalation, phonation, articulation, and resonance communicated by acoustic and auditory means.

These facile definitions serve only as pegs on which to hang a few of the numerous facets which are involved in complex human communication (Table 1.1).

How is this communicative system catered for in the development of human beings? Research shows that several modifications take place in different human organs to enable this development (Jesperson, 1922; DuBrul, 1958; Luchsinger and Arnold, 1965;

2

Table 1.1

Speech	Language
1. Productive	1. Perceptual
2. Mechanical	2. Cognitive
3. Motor (a) Neurophysiological (b) Neuromuscular	3. Neuropsychological
4. Components (a) breathing (b) phonation (c) resonance (d) articulation	4. Components (a) semantics (b) grammar (c) phonology (d) pragmatics

Denny-Brown, 1965; Lenneberg, 1967; Darley *et al.*, 1975; Kent, 1982, 1984).

THE VOCAL TRACT

The basic modification is that of the variation of timing imposed on output of air from the lungs. There are two major types of techniques of breathing, one for vital purposes and one for vocal purposes. To maintain life, human beings adopt a continual flow of breath, usually inhaling through the nose, taking air into the lungs in a rhythmic fashion and exhaling the breath again through the nose. To facilitate breathing for vocal purposes, a greater intake of air is usually made, the lungs are filled to greater capacity and the output of breath is more closely controlled to meet the needs of speech dictated by the length of utterance made. As in the case of vital breathing, this process is completely automatic and carried out with ease. For dramatic performances involving long speeches and soliloquies, actors make deliberate and conscious efforts to breathe more deeply and exert greater control on the out-going breath. Singers are also trained to use different forms of breathing and control. Such effort is not required in the course of normal conversational production. This is the fundamental evolutionary development employed to adapt a physical capacity primarily designed for one purpose, for use in another.

The primary function of the vocal folds, or cords, is that of protecting the lungs and their access, the tracheae, from the invasion of food and other foreign bodies. When considering studies of the vocal apparatus of man and of the great apes, Lenneberg (1967) notes that in several respects that of man is simpler:

> The geometry of the air spaces and fixed resonance chambers is 'streamlined'; there is only one set of functional vocal chords; the vocal chords are mounted in the air tunnel in such a way that, when adducted, they can produce sound only (or primarily) on expiration, instead of allowing both inspiratory and expiratory voice; and the epiglottis has moved so far below the pharynx as to allow the air from the larynx to stream freely through both nasal and oral cavities . . . it is precisely streamlining and simplification which, in many instances in animal morphology, constitute specialisation for given behaviour.
>
> (pp. 47–8)

The separation for vegetative purposes of the nasal and the oral cavities, by the movements of the soft palate and the action of the velo-pharyngeal sphincter, is a further advantageous feature for the development of speech. Variety of, and choice in, the variation of resonance relies to a great extent on this ability.

THE BRAIN

Study of cortical representation of the vocalization processes in the motor homunculus of the human brain, as described by Penfield and Rasmussen (1950), gives a clear indication of the importance of these organs and the need for them to be maintained in a healthy and active state. These authors noted that both mastication and swallowing are represented over a small area of the total which is concentrated on the organs concerned with vocalization and verbalization. Further, the organ most closely associated with the area of vocalization in the representation is the hand. The latter, of course, is widely involved in human communication. Manual dexterity is required for numerous language-linked activities, e.g. gesture (as in signing) and writing. The division of the area allotted to verbalization is also of interest. The greatest amount of cortical movement is concentrated upon the lips, followed by the jaw, the tongue and the face in that order. Swallowing and jaw movement show a similar amount of involvement. The bodily movement most closely related to that of vocalization is that of walking, with particular concentration on the movements of the knee, the ankle and the toes. These movements are all centred in the frontal lobes of the brain. The motor association area in the frontal lobes is also connected with integration and refinement of complex motor acts. But each cortico-cranial lobe is involved in the production of speech at some level or another.

Although both the right and left hemispheres are concerned in the reception, comprehension and production of language, there is overwhelming evidence that the left hemisphere of the human brain is dominant for all of those skills. Each hemisphere is comprised of four lobes. The following descriptions refer to the left hemisphere.

The occipital lobe

Starting from the rear of the cortex, the occipital lobe is the smallest of the four lobes of the brain and is concerned with vision and visual associations. The most significant aspect of this function with regard to language is its connection with the visual monitoring by the listener of the visible speech movements, facial expression and gestures of the speaker and, of course, reading. Specific physical problems may arise in a completely mechanical way to interfere with the ability to read, for example, nystagmus (rhythmic or undulating movements of the eyes) which may accompany some forms of dysarthria, and ocular dyspraxia (inability to carry out voluntary movements of the eyes on request). Both may interfere with the ability to concentrate on the written word. Thus neurophysiological visual skills are required to enable individuals to read. Reading is a symbolic aspect of language. Lesions may distort representations by several means and include different aspects of sight and recognition which, in turn, disrupt language use, e.g. visual perceptual dysfunctions such as colour agnosia, associative visual agnosia and pure word blindness.

The temporal lobe

This lobe contains the area which interprets the auditory input from the environment (Wernicke's area). That is, although there is bilateral representation of auditory inputs, the greater proportion of linguistic stimulus received from the speaker(s) via acoustic waves is conveyed through the right ear to the temporal lobe in the left hemisphere. This transition apparently takes place by means of conversion systems which transform the acoustic energy into mechanical, hydraulic and eventually electrochemical energy to facilitate neurological processing (Nation and Aram, 1977). These units of energy are conveyed by the auditory, 8th cranial, nerve, to the primary cortex of the temporal lobe in the left hemisphere. At some point in this process auditory patterns are transformed into phonetic patterns, which, in turn, are eventually decoded into phonological sequences. Lesions of the left temporal lobe, particularly in the posterior area, may be associated with deficits in phonemic hearing causing patients discriminatory difficulties with phonemes, e.g. /pa/ and /ba/ or /ta/ and /da/. This problem is often associated with other language difficulties.

The parietal lobe

This important lobe, situated above the temporal and occipital lobes and behind the frontal lobe is, like the others, represented in both hemispheres of the human brain. The parietal lobe in the left hemisphere functions as an integration area for on-going behaviour, a cerebral 'Spaghetti Junction'. Numerous complex symptomatologies may arise when lesions extend from and beyond the parietal lobe itself. The parietal lobe is described more for its disruptions than for normal functioning. Since the left parietal lobe deals with the perception of somatosensory events and then undertakes functions with spatial elements involved, it appears to be the information centre for most modalities. Lesions in the parietal lobes alter normal body sensations and spatial orientation and result in clumsy movements which affect the intelligibility of speech.

The frontal lobe

The frontal lobe of the left hemisphere is of greatest significance when studying the physical and motor aspects of speech (Broca's area). Further reference to the activities which activate speech movements must include the fact that there are interactions throughout the brain, extending from the cortex to the mid and lower levels and including pyramidal, extrapyramidal, cerebellar and reticular systems.

Darley *et al.* (1975) claim that there are six levels of brain activity involved in motor speech organization and describe them as follows.

1. The lowest level concerned with reflex actions, is the lower motor neurone and is clinically known as the bulbar area.
2. The second lowest level is the vestibular-reticular level. This gives rise to tracts which project to the lower motor neurone and its function is to regulate the reflex activity of the lower motor neurone.
3. The extrapyramidal third level comprises the basal ganglia and other related nuclear masses. It is involved in the automatic aspects of motor performance.
4. The highest purely motor level, the fourth, is in the cerebral motor cortex and is involved mostly with 'voluntary' movements – the upper motor neurone.
5. The cerebellum is the fifth level which controls equilibrium, and the accuracy of responses initiated at the four lower levels.
6. This is a pre-frontal level, which is also dependent on cortical arrangements. It is concerned with planning and programming all aspects of movement and is known as the conceptual programming level.

Kolb and Milner (1979) found that some patients with pre-frontal lesions found no difficulty when imitating single facial gestures, such as pursing lips, sticking out tongue or opening jaws wide. However, if asked to perform a sequence of such movements, significant impairment resulted. These workers also revealed that such patients found difficulty with pencil and paper exercises requiring a series of gestures, e.g. Porteus mazes. Problem solving of a general nature also causes confusion.

All of these levels will be discussed further later when considering the possible pathological breakdowns in the motor systems of the brain.

Although the left side of the human brain is regarded as being dominant for language and speech, in the majority of individuals there is evidence that the right hemisphere does have a role to play and that without the integrated action of both hemispheres successful language comprehension and production cannot take place. When discussing dichotic listening, Beaumont (1983) indicates that the majority of 'speech-like and language related stimuli are reported more accurately from the right ear if presented in dichotic pairs' (p. 210) (that is, crossing to the left hemisphere). He contrasts stimuli associated with left ear advantage as 'environmental sounds and "non-verbal vocal tract" '. He lists the former as a running tap, traffic etc. and the latter as coughs and grunts. These have the common factor of not being speech-like and this may have importance when considering the involvement of the right hemisphere.

Code (1987) indicates three areas of specific note which have to be included in studies of brain dominance and organization: sex, age and handedness. The following discussion reflects some of his points.

Sex

Results of studies of both normal and brain-disordered subjects support the view that language is more left hemisphere represented in males than in females, who appear to be more bilaterally represented (McGlone, 1978, 1983). Beaumont (1983) recognizes several problems in this area of study. As with other subject areas he suggests that it may be the case that only positive outcomes of research are reported and followed up and, in addition, numbers may be skewed in most cases as there is frequently a higher ratio of males to females in most clinical samples. No final conclusions can be drawn from the investigations to date as there continues to be much disagreement between the results reported (McGlone, 1983).

Age

The debate as to whether babies are born with brains already lateralized for language or whether they are bilateral at birth and develop towards a left hemisphere dominance has not yet been resolved. Basser (1962) observed that acquired dysphasia in children was both less severe than in adults and made a speedier recovery. He based those claims on the facts that, firstly, children's brains are not lateralized at an early age and that, in the second place, developing brain tissue has greater plasticity than that of the adult brain. Lenneberg (1967) based much of his work on these beliefs. He claimed that the cerebral hemispheres are equipotential for language in children and that damage to the left hemisphere would result in substantial compensation by the right hemisphere. Hemispherectomy studies which are based to a large extent on the traditional plasticity hypothesis have been largely supplanted by more recent studies, re-examinations of the originals and the claims made for them. For example, St James-Roberts (1981) has re-appraised the majority of hemispherectomy studies. He concludes that Basser's work was deficient in the quality of its reporting and that it relied too much on anecdotal evidence. Therefore, the resultant conclusions drawn from it by Lenneberg also become untenable. Moscovitch (1981), working at the Centre for Research in Human Development in Toronto, claims that before one year of age, damage to either hemisphere results in lower verbal and performance IQ. After one year of age, he concludes that only left hemisphere damage results in lower verbal and performance IQ.

Lenneberg's additional contention that language was fully developed by the early teens, c. 14;0, is also proving to be misleading although no firm evidence is available to the contrary. He seemed to be suggesting that around chronological age 14;0 handicapped children, e.g. children with Down's syndrome, underwent a form of language 'freezing' whereby the level of language acquired up to that point, possibly language showing two to ten years delay in development, remained static for the remainder of their lives. It is now known clinically that the reverse of this is true. Considerable developmental linguistic gains can be, and are, made across the whole human age spectrum. In fact studies have investigated the apparent language developmental stages recognizable in ageing (Emery, 1986).

Handedness

Research reveals close correlations between language and the cerebral control of motor skills. Kertesz and Hooper (1982) suggest that praxis and language share the same neural structures. Evidence exists which indicates that between 90% and 96% of the population are right handers with left hemisphere specialization for language (Rasmussen and Milner, 1977; Segalowitz and Bryden, 1983). In their detailed study, Rasmussen and Milner found that approximately 4% of right handers have right hemisphere specification for language, particularly for speech production. They state that 15% of left handers have right hemisphere specialization and 15% have bilateral representation. Figures produced by Segalowitz and Bryden agreed with this. In 1973, Sand and Taylor suggested decreasing left, and more mixed, handedness with increase in age. Conclusions arrived at by Hardyck and Petrinovitch (1977), after reviewing the literature to that date, indicated that dominant right handers with no family history of left handedness have the strongest left hemisphere lateralization and that most left handers with no family history are also left hemisphere specialized for language. Where there is positive family history of left handedness, left handers are most likely to have bilateral representation for language. The latter group show quicker recovery from brain damage with fewer lasting effects. Code (1987) points out that researchers have acknowledged that factors other than handedness alone, such as culture, environment and individual differences, must always be considered where lateralization and organization of brain function are concerned.

SPEECH PRODUCTION

Neonates are not physically equipped to speak. Immediately after birth babies' vocal tracts resemble more closely those of non-human primates than those of adult humans (DuBrul, 1977; Laitman and Crelin, 1976). The human vocal tract undergoes substantial changes during the first year of life to the extent that it is almost impossible to claim resemblance between phonetic categories in adults and infant sound productions. Kent (1984) contends that maturation imposes a 'progressively ascending level of central nervous system control over vocalisation and other behaviours' (p. R889). He claims that initially production and perception capabilities are largely separate but they become integrated within the first few months of life. At first it appears that infants, in turn-taking, will only increase their vocalizations, but that eventually infants' sound productions reflect those of the adults around them (Stein et al., 1975). Studies of infants' productive behaviour may indicate that certain perceptual propensities may direct phonetic development to some degree. Research reveals that a cyclic tendency develops in human maturation (Kugler et al., 1980). Rhythm appears to play a major role in early vocal development, for example, in the repeated use of reduplicated babbling such as 'da da da'. This tendency is found in rhythmic body movements of the trunk, the limbs and the digits. It is interesting to note that in normal development these movements decrease around seven to eight months when babbling becomes the greatest preoccupation of the child. Thelen (1981) proposed that rhythmic stereotypes, as he called them, are the transition between uncoordinated and coordinated movements, and act as a preparatory stage between the two. This reflects to some degree the claims that Piaget (1956) made for the importance of rhythm as a stage in cognitive development, particularly in the form of repetition (e.g. in primary, secondary and tertiary circular reactions observed in the sensorimotor period). Kent (1984) postulates that:

> Rhythmic movements in speech and in other motor systems may contribute to (i) an infant's discovery of optimal timing control or kinesiological efficiency and, (ii) the development of coordination within and among motor systems . . . the fact that reduplicated babbling occurs together with peak frequencies of rhythmic stereotypes in other parts of the body indicates . . . that reduplicated babbling is perhaps not a limited phonological process but rather a part of a more general developmental process in which cyclicity is used to motor advantage. Indeed rhythmic stereotypes may be a first major sign of the emergence of coordination.
>
> (p. R892)

Kent goes on to suggest that the infant's early coding of speech is different from that of the adult. For example, units of phonological contrast appear to be larger in the early stages of language acquisition than those of the adult language user. In fact it has been proposed that in early sound development, the units of phonological contrast are syllables and words and not phonemes,

11

as is presumably the case with adults. Thus it can be claimed that the acquisition of phonology interacts with the acquisition of motor control for speech. The child certainly requires the skill to manipulate the vocal tract for the production of individual sounds and to arrange the movements of the muscles to produce sound sequences. Alternatively, praxis for articulation relies to some degree on the emergence of phonetic contrasts and demands made for the production of long sound sequences. On-going development of precision of movement and increase of lexicon by the child, accompanied by improving self-monitoring skills, leads to the establishment of a reliable, intelligible and automatic productive speech system.

Development of normal praxis for speech production

In the course of an investigation to identify and assess developmental articulatory dyspraxia (DAD) (Milloy, 1985) it became necessary to set up a small survey to determine the age by which normally developing children established praxis for articulation, i.e., when their motor skills reached the stage of automatic movement to enable them to produce reliable articulation on each attempt at production. Thirty-five children were longitudinally observed and assessed over a period of four years during which their ages ranged from 3;0 to 7;0. The mean age for the development of motor skills for articulation was calculated as 6;0. The children were assessed on the Edinburgh Articulation Test (EAT) (Anthony et al., 1971) and the experimental version of the Milloy Assessment of Praxis (MAP). The results agreed with those of Kools and Tweedie (1975), who found that normally developing children establish praxis for limb and oral movements by age 6; 0. A further finding resulting from Milloy's study indicated that in the population of children with moderate learning disabilities the majority, i.e. around 90%, show evidence of immature praxis in their articulatory as well as in their general motor skills. This maturational delay affects language and will be discussed later. Children with severe learning disabilities are, of course, proportionately more severely affected in all motor skills and as a result of this frequently develop deviant language forms.

Research is beginning to indicate greater understanding of the motor milestones acquired by children as they develop towards adult independence. However, little is known of how children build up coordinated actions or which environmental conditions are most conducive to their development. Similarly, there is a paucity of information on the strategies children use to establish the ability to sequence movements and acquire accuracy of spatial localization in motor performance. It seems reasonable to assume that awareness of results of action and repetition, by trial and error, of serially ordered movements will lead to the ability to monitor and repair. Observation of the reduction of redundant movements and the selection of laterality in the course of repeated actions indicates that motor memories are being developed and that inhibition is being employed to curtail extraneous movements. Kent (1981), discussing the development of the vocal tract, stated that the presence of a normal vocal tract did not completely determine output, nor did it guarantee the development of normal speech. Sharkey and Folkins (1985) devised a study to measure variability of lip and jaw movements in children and adults. They used groups of five adults, and children aged 4;0, 7;0 and 10;0, who produced [mae] and [bae] 20 times each. The duration of lip-opening movements, jaw-opening movements, lip-open postures, jaw-open postures and the timing between the onset of lower lip opening and jaw opening decreased in variability between the child and the adult groups. Significant results were recorded in a decrease of variability of lower lip displacement between the 4;0 and 7;0 year age groups. No other significant results were forthcoming. It was hypothesized that different developmental motor processes affect the variability of speech movements at early, intermediate and older ages.

CRITICAL/SENSITIVE PERIODS OF LEARNING

Embryologists were probably the first researchers to suggest the existence of apparent critical periods for acquiring certain stages in development in man. As with numerous aspects of human development the realization of this fact followed the study of abnormal development. For example, the occurrence of cleft palate results, in most cases, from the failure of fusion of the palatal plates which form the hard palate. It is known that in the course of normal development this fusion occurs at some time between 12 and 16 weeks of foetal development. Therefore it can be assumed that this four week period is critical for palatal development. Later, psychologists realized that it was possible that children acquired certain behaviours when there is a state of readiness prevailing for the specific development of such behaviours. Lorenz (1961) has described the imprinting of young birds as being a critical period which takes place only during a brief interval after hatching. It is debatable as to whether a parallel can be drawn between the imprinting of young birds and periods of sensitivity in human beings. It is claimed by Lenneberg, (1967) that there is a critical period for the acquisition of language. Again this was claimed from studies of recovery of language after injury (i.e. from the abnormal standpoint) to the left hemisphere of the brain. Later writers have disputed this particular aspect as a claim for critical period learning. However, Ritchie *et al.* (1975) state that while the adult brain is remarkably resistant, the developing brain is critically vulnerable. They also mention the period which is developmentally most critical of all – the 'growth spurt' between 2 to 3 months before birth to 2 years after birth, and the fact that an adult/child dyad is required for brain growth in infancy. Netsell (1981) says that embryogenesis and other fetal developments represent 'critical periods' in the infant's maturation. He goes on to state that:

Sensitive periods of nonlinearity occur when certain neural, musculoskeletal, environmental and cognitive changes combine (or 'get together') in the individual organism. The points in time at which a particular number of these factors combine can result in 'jumps in performance' that appear incremental if not placed on a conceptually broader map of sensorimotor and cognitive development.

(p. 136)

Dobbing (1972) points out that not only have many behavioural aspects of individual behaviour to be acquired at certain times during the period shortly after birth, but also some of the later growth processes in the brain are vulnerable. He emphasizes the nutritional factors involved. Malnutrition before or shortly after birth in human infants can have a lasting effect on, for example, mental development. Mounting evidence is available that permanent deficits can be produced by various forms of interference with behavioural development during early, vulnerable periods. The speech therapist is aware of this fact in the observation of specific speech and/or language disabilities which persist and frequently defy treatment. Reference will be made to these at a later stage.

Motoi speech control

It appears that speech, the physical production of language, is also subject to critical period influence. The acquisition of language, including its spoken aspects, is dependent on the shared ability of the speaker and the listener, each of whom is programmed to develop a similar system based on the language components available to all human beings and the mother tongue of the country of origin. The situation is made easier by the fact that each individual is both speaker and listener, on different occasions. Although this book is concerned with speech primarily, reference has to be made to those aspects of language which constitute the message, or response which has to be conveyed by what Fry (1977) calls 'the complex machinery for speech which we possess' (p. 20). Language has its beginnings in the infant's ability to select its various signals from the mass of signals surrounding him/her. Studies report that there is a period during which this process begins (Stark *et al.*, 1975; Crystal, 1979). Thus the assumption can be made that in the case of normally developing infants there is a sensitive period during which this initiation into the medium of language takes place. The timing for this occurrence is around 2 to 3 months. The form this takes is of the child's awareness of prosodic contrasts in the adult language directed at her/him. Although the human infant begins to use speech forms at an early stage, they are indiscriminate. Vocalizations practised by the child assume first resemblances to the mother tongue at around 6 months of age. This, therefore, is another critical period of learning, and the first expression of meaningful use of the mother tongue.

Infants throughout the world share linguistic and motor universals, not least of which seems to be the timing device by which continuing skills are facilitated and learned. This has important implications for teachers and therapists and will be discussed at length at a later stage. However, language will only be learned in an atmosphere conducive to learning. This necessitates an adult/child dyad in which the adult enables the child, by means of frequent repetition and clearly delivered speech, to listen to a good language model and also makes it possible for the child to practise turn-taking as used in normal conversation. Healthy, normal children acquire the habit of language relatively quickly and usually painlessly. Even in adverse circumstances, children developing normally acquire speech. It is only in cases of disability that the process becomes burdensome and fraught with difficulties. Through the analysis of the breakdown of language, investigators can better understand by what means language has been acquired in the first place.

2

Genetic conditions and structural deviations

The following chapters describe conditions which interfere with the normal acquisition of speech. Examples of such conditions are divided into three major areas of breakdown: genetic, structural and neurological. It should be noted that in this context *genetic* refers to deviations and aberrations in the genetic code and type of the individual. Both structural and neurological defects and/or deficits may have an inherited factor, but this is a different aspect of genesis. Each of these areas will be subjected to scrutiny from three viewpoints: description; development, including effects of speech and language development; and speech therapy management.

GENETIC CONDITIONS

Description

Every human cell contains a necklace-like strand of 46 non-solid threads which constitute the chemistry of the individual's heredity. These are chromosomes. In turn, each chromosome comprises around 50 000 genes, every one carrying a vital piece of information necessary to produce a complete, new human being. Each parent contributes 23 chromosomes. With one exception these chromosomes are well matched from the parents' stores of chromosomes. The exception is the 'odd man out' male sex, or Y chromosome. The female sex chromosome, the X chromosome, appears to be the more stable and is possibly the factor for the longer survival of females, and other signs of female stability.

There is evidence that one or other of the sex chromosomes features significantly in many deviant conditions (DHSS, 1972). Genes can mutate spontaneously or through the effect of drugs, radiation or other factors. Genetic counselling has become a reliable means of explanation and prediction for numerous families. Basic gene structure is better understood all the time, and researchers are uncovering numerous factors which enable the medical profession not only to treat, but also to prevent serious defects in succeeding generations.

It is recognized that familial diathesis is of paramount importance, although the trigger to eventual effects may often be environmental. For example, in Leicester, the recorded incidence by speech therapists of child stutterers fell dramatically during the 1960s, and it was not until the appearance of a remarkable number of stutterers among the families of Asian immigrants that the possibility was considered that the more permissive attitudes of British parents in that decade removed the pressures which had previously resulted in triggering stuttering in children predisposed to stutter. The parents in the ethnic community placed very high expectations on their children, educationally and culturally, and possibly exerted sufficient constraints to activate stuttering in the children predisposed to it.

On British television (BBC) an experiment is being monitored by geneticists on a large family in which several members have different speech and/or language disorders, i.e. familial diathesis (Antennae, 1989). The aim is to isolate the 'gene for speech'.

Developmental associations

Genetically determined congenital abnormalities can affect all aspects of development – motor, sensory, perceptual intellectual, emotional and behavioural. In addition to the anatomical, physiological and neurological deviations from the norm which occur in the presence of an abnormal genotype, there appears to be slowed or unequal growth and acquisition of skills, both physical and mental. One aspect of this developmental impedance is manifested in the acquisition of communication skills which themselves rely on the normal, healthy development of a child.

Consider the effects of a genetic problem on the development of a specific child by referring to *Down's syndrome*, which is the most common chromosomal abnormality. This occurs in two recognizable forms. The more common is the non-disjunction defect which accounts for 95% of cases, and in which the older mother is increasingly at risk. There is some evidence that the paternal age may also be relevant (Cunningham, 1982). Translocation is the second type, and is responsible for 5% of children with Down's syndrome (DS) born to young mothers. The incidence is 1 : 1600 in women of less than 20 years of age, and the former 1 : 75 in women of more than 40 years of age. The clinical features of both types are identical. For the purposes of this book the features of greatest interest are those affecting speech. There is one vital feature which is not yet fully accepted. The child with DS usually has microcephaly. This indicates that the head and all it accommodates will be affected by the reduction in skull size. The tongue is usually of normal dimensions. This fact influences the management of the case and will be discussed later. The most frequently presenting oral defects are as follows:

1. palate, narrow and foreshortened;
2. small nose, depressed nasal bridge;
3. under-developed teeth;
4. tendency for tongue to furrow with age.

In addition, there is chronic mouth-breathing, accompanying frequent upper respiratory tract infections, and a strong likelihood of intermittent conductive hearing loss.

There is a well-documented history of language delay, although it was thought that the development of language followed normal stages but at a markedly retarded rate (Lenneberg, 1967). More recent work on the acquisition of particular language structures disputes this claim and indicates that DS children are significantly weaker than retarded, but non-DS children at sequential and syntactic processing (Hartley, 1982). Cunningham et al. (1985) claim that children with DS show increasing language delay with age, and they note that this is more evident in boys than girls. One study (Stoel-Gammon, 1980) indicates that the phonological development of children demonstrates that they develop phonologies similar to those of normally developing children, but at a retarded rate, and that they favour particular positions within words.

19

Management

Before proceeding to describe the management recommended for the production of speech in the DS population it is necessary to clarify some important points. This work has set out to expand upon speech therapy specifically in the field of speech. Careful distinctions have to be made between language disorders and speech disorders in this context (Table 1.1). Although speech, or articulation disorders, are the prime concern here, it cannot be emphasized strongly enough that language and speech intervention should be undertaken simultaneously. The contention on which this work is based is that the physical, mechanical and basic first stages of speech and expressive language readiness have recently been neglected. In some cases this neglect has been total, with the result that advanced language therapy has been undertaken with children who are neither physically nor spatially/temporally in a state of readiness to succeed at such levels. Such a child may be attempting to produce three or four word utterances, but be in a perpetual state of open-mouthed stuffiness, possibly accompanied by a greater or lesser degree of fluctuating conductive deafness and therefore in a poor position to reach her/his potential linguistically.

It is strongly recommended that the role of the speech therapist includes being an enabler to direct and counsel the parent(s) in how to help the child to reach a level of physical receptiveness to allow her/him to utilize her/his speech organs most effectively. The basic steps available to achieve this state will, hereafter, be referred to as the basic exercises (BE) (Appendix A).

BE enhances the skills which are fundamental to the production of speech and, in the case of normally developing children, these become automatic at a very early stage. Without this foundation, all later and more complex skills will be adversely affected and goals set will prove much more difficult to attain. Children with DS will not find the acquisition of such skills either easy or motivating, so it is also necessary to stimulate interest in their achievement. Parents will usually be well motivated to succeed with such exercises, as they welcome anything which will help their child to appear more 'normal'. It is essential to ensure that parents themselves can successfully carry out the exercises which the child is expected to perfect!

A study reported by Southall *et al.* (1987) describes a condition previously undetected, in which some children with DS evince severe upper airway obstruction which can be partial or complete. Choanal dilation and/or surgery for the removal of infected tonsils or overgrown adenoids helped in a few cases. Application of the learned control of the above techniques for breathing and the maintenance of clear nasal passageways may reduce the possibility of this alarming situation. Means should be sought to find the easiest form of practice for each child. It is recommended that the BE should be carried out at least twice each day and more often where possible. Most of the exercises can be made either a source of fun or an interesting part of everyday living.

There are characteristic forms of speech disabilities in the DS population. These include dysarthria and its accompanying disorders of resonance; specific articulatory problems; dysfluency and particular types of voice disorder which will also affect resonance. Management has to be tailored to the needs of the individual and usually has to be planned within the limits of attention, concentration and application. It is infinitely better to approach all these problems in a pragmatic context. For example, the child should be helped to understand how best to meet needs, indicate desires and express feelings within her/his idiosyncratic limitations. The appreciation of turn-taking, eye-contact, awareness of gesture and body language and some repair techniques may be learned in play situations. This will only succeed if the parents understand the significance of such aspects of communication.

The Russian school's theory of the directive function of speech is one of the best means of practising the use of expressive language (Luria and Yudovich, 1971). More recently, conductors working with severely physically handicapped children at the Institute for the Motor Disabled in Budapest have referred to this interaction between the mental and physical attribut s of learning as 'rhythmic intention' (Harri and Tillemans, 1984). By this means, every action, every intention, in fact every thought is expressed aloud by the child in the course of carrying out all the activities of everyday living. It may be that this method imposes too great a strain on the capabilities of the majority of children with DS, but it is worth practising for at least part of each day, to improve the dysarthric condition and upgrade intelligibility. When dealing with the most severely speech handicapped children, it may be necessary to implement an alternative and/or augmentative communicative system, such as Makaton (Le Prevost, 1983).

21

Consider carefully the environmental aspects of the person with DS when planning alleviation for voice problems. After the physical conditions of the individual have been improved there sometimes remains a situation in which vocal abuse, caused by shouting, is perpetuated in the home or ward either as a means of 'keeping one's end up' or as a specific symptom of dysarthria caused by lack of control of vocal volume. Diplomatic counselling may improve the former. Prosodic therapy may have to be used to deal with uncontrolled loudness. The concept of one-to-one treatment for people with DS is no longer appropriate when planning speech and/or language therapy. Experience indicates that good modelling, careful timing, meaningful discourse and sufficient practice added to optimum physical conditions are the most effective means of enabling improvement in this type of client. The best way of implementing communication appears to be by group therapy in which the children and their parents are encouraged to interact with each other in learning simple concepts of space, time, size, number, colour and so on. If an augmentative system of communication is introduced it is imperative that parents, teachers, playgroup leaders and all concerned adults are taught to use it in a consistent fashion so that confusion may be avoided and open communication channels surround the child.

Parent groups have proved invaluable in many different ways. For example, there is the initial need of parents themselves to 'work out' their particular problems by discussion with others in similar circumstances. Most parents find it difficult to appreciate that many others share the, apparently overwhelming, problems which arise from trying to rear a disabled child. Until this point has been acknowledged, many parents are unable either to share their anxieties with others, or to give of their best to the child who needs their constant attention. A vital factor in this context is to realize that society no longer expects them to carry the burden alone. Nor is it felt that they, the parents, must sacrifice their whole lives to the care of their handicapped child, but that they are entitled to have a life of their own. Gradually, both parents themselves and society as a whole are becoming able to apportion responsibility for the future of disabled children.

There is a trend at present for some parents of DS children to seek surgery in an attempt to make their children look more acceptable. This is a choice which all parents may exercise. Two points arise here. Firstly, there is no evidence to suggest the long-term success of such intervention. In the second place, surgery only changes outward appearances. Personal, social and cognitive abilities are unaltered. The child with DS is accepted by present day society because he/she is easily identifiable by his/her appearance. If the appearance is changed, society will expect his/her behaviour to change and this will not happen. The child may then be in an even less secure position than originally. Other disabled or handicapped children whose appearance is more like that of their 'normal' contemporaries may suffer more in that they are expected to function at higher levels than it may be possible for them to reach. This could be the fate of children with DS after surgery. Having previously claimed that individuals with DS have a normal-sized tongue within a reduced-sized mouth it would seem that tongue-reduction surgery is probably counter-productive and may, in fact, reduce a child's ability to control his/her articulatory movements. Other forms of surgery available include nasal bridge improvement, reduction of epicanthic folds and division of syndactylic digits. There is no evidence that any of these interventions improve the state of the DS child, or indeed are permanent physical modifications.

Examples of other types of genetically transmitted conditions which affect speech include, for example, *fragile-X syndrome*, *muscular dystrophy*, and *Klinefelter's syndrome*. Individual needs have to be met in an attempt to improve and/or remediate each of these. Many syndromes of a genetic nature result in children being so severely handicapped that they grow up mentally retarded or do not survive. If the former, it usually means that normal language is never fully acquired and speech is limited in its production.

To some extent, there is an element of genetic influence in all types of deviance, and it could be claimed that every constellation of symptoms found in children with developmental problems derives from inherited factors. However, a distinction has to be made between those conditions which result from blatant chromosomal aberrations and mutations, and those which result from a triggering of predisposing factors, for example, the incidence of stuttering mentioned above. Changing attitudes are influencing the basic philosophy in the training of speech therapists and there tends to be less thought of 'treatment' and more of facilitating 'learning'. In addition, with the implementation of findings such as those arrived at by the Warnock commission (1979) and particularly its recommendation that where possible children should be educated in mainstream schools and thus integrated into society at an early age, a step has been taken to enable such children to attain their learning potentials. Unfortunately, due to financial shortfalls and recent cutbacks, there has been no opportunity either to train teachers in mainstream schools to deal with these children's specific needs, or to reduce class numbers to ensure that no child, either normal or slow-learning, suffers as a result. Forward planning is not a strong point of our British society.

STRUCTURAL DEVIATIONS

Description

Numerous conditions may arise as a result of the maldevelopment or deformity of those parts of the vocal tract on which speech is dependent. For instance, the tongue, lips, palate, pharyngeal and laryngeal organs are all prone to various defects. Some of these will be described in more detail later in the discussion of structural deviations.

The most devastating type of oral cavity fault is that of the cleft palate anomalad. This defect, like all others to which the human being is liable, can manifest itself as mild, moderate or severe in degree. In essence, the cleft palate anomalad may be regarded as being primarily of a genetic nature; it is also one of the most damaging of structural deviations that may affect the speech apparatus of a human infant. In cases of mild involvement, only a unilateral cleft of the upper lip may be present. At the other end of the scale, bilateral clefts may split both sides of the lip and the hard and soft palates affecting the total surfaces of tissue from front to back and depriving the child of any useful division between the oral and nasal cavities. In such cases the prime need to be met is that of feeding for survival, and methods should be found to facilitate this.

Developmental association

The speech therapist may be recruited to help and advise nursing staff and parents with feeding. His/her role may be to recommend that the orthodontist should examine the infant to decide whether a prosthesis should be made to facilitate sucking and swallowing (Selley and Boxall, 1986). In addition, there may be reduced use of the tip of the tongue during feeding. Thus, screening of the movements of the tongue tip should be an early assessment. Several orthodontic appliances are available to facilitate feeding, while at the same time protecting the exposed mucosa and attempting to align the cleft segments of the lips and alveolus (Gornall *et al.*, 1983). Despite their severe physical deformities, many babies with cleft palate manage to feed reasonably well with a normal bottle and teat. It is important to position the baby properly to prevent choking. He/she should be held in a partially elevated position resting on the lap. Brookshire *et al.* (1980) recommend that babies should be allowed to set their own pace when feeding. Such a baby may require longer and more frequent feeding times pre-surgery. Haberman (1988) describes the problems she experienced with feeding her daughter born with *Pierre Robin Syndrome*, a congenital abnormality in which the child has a very small lower jaw, posterior cleft palate and an abnormally placed tongue retracted towards the pharyngeal space, known as glossoptosis; this condition can render breathing difficult and impossible in severe cases. After trial-and-error attempts with numerous feeding appliances her baby had to be tube-fed in order to survive. Necessity motivated Haberman to try out alternative methods of feeding and consequently she was successful using a dummy and a syringe. Later, she made a more sophisticated version which is now commercially available. Whatever method of feeding is used, it is essential to clean out the mouth thoroughly after each feed and be sure that the whole area is cleared of all food.

Parents usually have to be helped to relax and to aim to enable the child to enjoy both the feed and the close proximity of the parent. If this is carried out in the right order, everyone will benefit and on the rare occasion when the child may choke, there will be no tendency to panic. Furthermore, parents should still be expected to talk to their babies during feeding and to give them the chance to feel part of the dyad, twosome, which is so important in the learning process.

The custom in the UK is to carry out early surgical intervention in cases of cleft palate. This is done expressly to obviate the possibility of the child developing disordered articulation and resonance due to the malformation and malapproximation of the different areas within the mouth and pharynx. In most cases surgery is completely successful and the development of the child's speech is normal. Where some problems remain, they usually take the form of small fistulae along the line of the repair to the palate. This will seldom affect articulation and is much more likely to distort resonance. Resultant speech may be hypernasal and, in severe cases, intelligibility is affected. Speech therapy can often resolve the problem quite quickly (see pp. 123–8).

Other areas involved in the development of children with cleft palate frequently depend on different factors pertaining in their genotypical makeup. As with all children, there will be the very able, those of average ability and the less able. Similarly, there will be some in the group with degrees of clumsiness of movement while others have normal motor skill abilities.

Management

Children with speech defects resulting from the effects of cleft palate should be assessed as soon as possible to permit early intervention. As previously stated, steps should be taken to facilitate as near-normal feeding habits as can be achieved in the presence of either the distortion of oral space created by the cleft or the disrupted forms of tissue resulting from the surgery. Optimal physical condition should be the aim. Speech therapy can do a great deal to improve this situation and diagnostic therapy should be followed which includes every effort to improve palatal movement in all possible positions. In the small number of instances where this method fails, the speech therapist may have to refer the child back to the medical team for secondary surgery, such as pharyngoplasty, before starting on speech therapy. Only when the best possible state of the mechanism has been attained can a programme of management be activated.

All aspects of language, speech and hearing should be assessed. Many children born with clefts of the palate have been discovered to have coexisting language disabilities affecting one or more components of language, other than phonology which it would be expected would be involved. Development of phonology will be distorted due to the absence of reliable phonetic patterns of production on which to build the system. As a result, syntax, morphology and sometimes semantics will be affected to a greater or lesser degree. Some cases will present with problems confined only to the phonetic and phonological aspects of language, and yet others may have articulation and phonological disorders co-occurring, the latter often due to some form of hearing loss.

Relatively frequently, children with repaired palates have a history of car infection and/or eustachian tube blockages (glue ear) resulting from craniofacial damage to the middle third of the face so crucial for the acceptable production of speech. Where both language and speech are defective the therapist will have to decide which constitutes the priority for each individual. In the majority of cases, both aspects usually have to be included in management planning, although it may be possible for the speech therapist to incorporate the help of the parent, playgroup or class teacher to provide the modelling and backup for the language deficits, while in clinic she concentrates on the mechanical difficulties.

Expressive language can only succeed where the anatomical, physiological and neurological systems can support it. The speech therapist's remit includes administering the required assessments. These could be, for example, a progress checklist such as that of Gerard (1985), the revised Reynell Developmental Language Scale (RDLS) (1985) to screen for general language use, the Language Assessment, Remediation and Screening Procedure (LARSP) (1976), the Profile in Semantics (PRISM) (1982) and phonological analysis of cleft palate speech (Lynch *et al.*, 1983; Grunwell and Russell, 1988). The battery employed to assess the functional status of the vocal tract should include checks on breathing techniques and breath control, phonation, resonance and prosody with particular emphasis on velopharyngeal sphincter competence. Albery *et al.* (1986) recommend diagnostic therapy for children with 'total glottal stop pattern'. The Edinburgh Articulation Test (EAT) should be used to determine both the quantitative and qualitative nature of the speech. At the same time this assessment will indicate the measure of immaturity which may be present, and which may have to be considered when making long-term treatment programmes.

The speech therapist is also responsible for the reduction of nasal escape as already stated. This may result from the persistence of small fistulae along the line of the repair to the palate. More often it is a result of an insufficient velopharyngeal seal. Articulation may be affected by the absence of central or lateral incisors. This affects the maintenance of the central airstream required for sibilant fricatives, /s/ and /z/, and lateralization may develop. Resonance becomes distorted. Resultant speech will be hypernasal and, in severe cases, intelligibility is affected. Speech therapy can resolve this problem quite quickly. Intervention may take the following form:

1. Enable the child to *hear* the difference between *oral* and *nasal* speech.
   (a) Select a short phrase with no nasal consonants in it, e.g. 'here's teddy', and repeat it on audiotape.
   (b) Play it to child and ask him/her to repeat it several times.
   (c) Say the phrase once more and audiotape the child repeating it several times.
   (d) Play back the two performances until the child *hears* the difference.
2. Enable the child to *feel* the difference between *oral* and *nasal* speech.
   (a) Use two cards, about one third of postcard size, on each of which is placed a piece of tissue paper (cut in the shape of a teddy, if desired). Demonstrate what happens when the breath is expired, first down the nose and then out of the mouth, while one card is held just under the nose and the second is held just under the lower lip. Repeat until the child *feels* the difference.
   (b) With the cards still in position, repeat the phrases 'here's teddy' and 'mummy's coming' until the child *feels* the difference while using speech.
3. Enable the child to *see* the difference between *oral* and *nasal* speech.
   (a) Repeat the above exercise holding, instead of cards with tissue paper, two small mirrors, in the positions described. Demonstrate by repeating /t/, /t/, /t/ then /ŋ/, /ŋ/, /ŋ/ to illustrate that only the mirror held under the lower lip mists over in the production of the former, and only the mirror held under the nose mists over in the production of the latter.
   (b) With the mirrors still in position, repeat the phrases 'here's teddy' and 'mummy's coming' until the child *sees* the difference while using speech.

The child should now be able to distinguish between *hearing*, *seeing* and *feeling* the *oral* and *nasal* direction of breath in speech. Practising such approaches to reduce or eliminate nasal escape by using voluntary movements may enable the child eventually to automatize the movements. It is essential that such exercises are undertaken before working on specific production patterns. The child should be encouraged to self-monitor to ensure that the correct breath directions are maintained. Different forms of instrumentation are available for this purpose such as the anemometer, the micronose and the 'N' indicator all of which provide visual evidence of nasal escape.

Russell (1989) sets the following therapeutic objectives:

1. encourage a widening range of speech-like vocalizations at both pre- and speech stages;
2. participate in babbling and imitation with visual stimulation and exaggerated movements;
3. instruct parent in those speech-like sounds which should be discouraged, e.g. glottal plosives;
4. demonstrate tactile stimulation to parent, e.g. mother places finger against child's mouth during vocalization; child's hand taken to mother's mouth;
5. incorporate the use of face crayons; make-up; licking spoon with suitable food;
6. auditory and discrimination skills, e.g. telephone bell, animal noises, consonant identification;
7. consonant drill;
8. games to encourage recognition of pragmatic language including aspects presenting greatest difficulty.

Group, as well as individual, intervention is discussed by Brookshire *et al.* (1980). They recommend integrated therapeutic objectives involving natural interaction between children with similar productive problems. It is much more realistic to encourage children to interact with and relate to each other in circumstances which are familiar to them and which they are likely to face in everyday contexts. Also, each child's individual experience will equip her/him to share problems which arise in a group as well as enabling the children to learn from each other. It is also useful for children with cleft palate speech to be included in groups in which children with other but similar types of language/speech disorders interact.

Discussing management, Albery and Russell (1990) emphasize the need for:

1. careful assessment;
2. intervention for velopharyngeal insufficiency;
3. investigating auditory discrimination;
4. investigating recognition by the child of her/his errors in both the clinician's and his/her own speech;

5. investigating the child's ability to produce correctly all deviant consonants in both isolation and combinations;
6. establishing 'new' consonants in different syllable and word positions.

These writers also underlined the greater improvements which accrue from intensive therapy than from extended periods of weekly therapy.

Parents in the UK have derived a great deal of help from the Cleft Lip and Palate Parents' Association (CLAPPA), which enables them to visit and counsel each other. Much benefit issues from sharing problems and discussing means of supporting their children, as well as devising methods to ease situations which arise in school, for example, compensatory means of enabling the most severely affected children to deal with feeding difficulties. The speech therapists' Infants at Risk Group also helps parents.

Other physical conditions which interfere with the development include the Pierre Robin Syndrome, already mentioned. Although this frequently involves cleft palate, it does not always do so. However, articulation may be affected as it is the head and face which are involved. The salient factor is the retrognathic mandible, or small chin. About 30% of children with this syndrome have learning disabilities and the majority have articulation disorders arising from the restricted oral space and the tongue position. Compensatory articulatory placements are often possible and allow for different degrees of intelligibility. Traditional articulation therapy, in which practice of sounds in isolation, in syllables, in words and phrases and finally in sentences is only useful initially with cases which have been assessed for both sensorimotor oral awareness and an intact ability to self-monitor. Almost invariably it will be necessary to use BE (see Appendix A, p. 142) to adjust poor breathing patterns and introduce self-controlled oral/nasal hygiene. Assessment of oral sensory awareness can then be determined as follows:

1. awareness of total oral space – from front to back, from lower to upper perimeters and from side to side;
2. awareness of different textures – sharpness, even and uneven surfaces (teeth), concave, convex, hard, soft, static, mobile;
3. awareness of temperature, pressure, breath direction (nasal and oral) and sound direction (nasal and oral), vibration from tongue and lip movements.

This whole area should be assessed prior to specific articulatory practice.

The first stage of this programme is designed to draw to the child's attention the sensations and effects of movement within the mouth cavity. Phonetic production relies on flexibility of the organs of speech, precise, clean, fast movements and reliable sensory feedback-loop systems. By discussion, demonstration and shared participation the child, or a group of children, and the clinician can identify the positions and approximations of, for example, the lips in the production of /b/ and /m/ and the tip of the tongue and the alveolar ridge in the production of /t/ and /n/. For discrimination of front, middle and back of the oral cavity and the segments that are produced at each position, see page 63, and the reference to Klick (1985). Exaggerated movements of the tongue along the cheeks can be observed and imitated in shared mirror work as can be all types of lip movement. Concept training is sometimes required to facilitate the understanding of *front/middle/back*, *behind/in front*, *up/down* and other contrasts. *Right* and *left* may present considerable problems and not until these are established, or at least brought to full awareness and compensated for, will the child be able to succeed with the task (Frostig and Horne, 1966). This is primarily a positional/visual, spatial/temporal experience, rather than a linguistic one.

As previously stated, children with speech/language disorders frequently cannot identify themselves in time and space. Part of this problem leads to their inability to fully understand specific words which describe spatial and temporal situations. Experience indicates that relatively frequently children attempt to carry out instructions about which they have little or no comprehension, and also that after a concept has been established it may continue to include learned errors, e.g. 'I wented to school tomorrow' Fraser and Blockley (1973) describe a child with delayed language development reported by his speech therapist to be making no progress and referred to them for psychological assessment. On the discovery that the child had no stable knowledge of himself in space and time, he was instructed in this area. Results included the eventual acquisition and development of language without further intervention after the child had worked out his own physical place in his world.

To fulfil the requirements of the second stage, considerable time should be spent in exploring and improving proprioceptive and tactile awareness by moving the tongue and the finger around within the mouth to identify parts, their dimensions, their textures and their particular characteristics. Once more, preliminary screening will ascertain whether the child is *au fait* with the terms being used for this purpose. It is probable that children who have recently benefited from BE will have become aware of the different 'feeling' within their mouths created by the new juxtaposition of the jaws, which will now be approximated, bringing the upper and lower surfaces into unaccustomed contact. This should facilitate numerous experiments with all possible permutations which can be performed by various movements of the jaws, lips, velum and tongue.

The third stage involves, for example, raising the tongue within the mouth and wiggling it backwards and forwards, repeating the movement with the tongue outside the mouth. The object of this is to contrast the feeling of the tongue when it is *warm* inside the mouth and *cold* outside the mouth. Similar temperature changes can be experienced when the blade of a spoon is held under cold water then gently inserted inside the mouth along the surface of the tongue. This is repeated after the spoon has been held under warm water. Appreciation of these sensitive distinctions enables the child to increase sensory experience and improve awareness which may not have been well stimulated during the period when the child's mouth was habitually open, preventing such changes in temperature. Another use of the blade of the spoon can emphasize changes in pressure in the mouth. Being careful to avoid causing the child to gag, the tongue can be depressed by the spoon, first near the front and then further back.

Practice of the exercise to differentiate between nasal and oral expiration may also be useful (see page 28). Sound direction is dependent on the use of nasal v. oral consonants. Games can be designed to introduce competition into the situation. Humming on /m/ will heighten the sensitivity level of the lips, while trilling on /r/ will create a similar sensation in the tongue. Such exercises will enable children to replace the articulatory muscular experience and sensory awareness which they apparently missed out on in the course of normal development. Treatment should now proceed to the use of comparisons and experiments with actual pronunciation patterns.

Establishment of reliable patterns of articulation will, in turn, provide the reliable feedback for self-monitoring so essential for the development of child phonologies. Hence, such therapy facilitates the natural basis for phonology advocated by Harris and Cottam (1985).

As can be seen, children occasionally require help to reach the level of *physical readiness* needed to develop an acceptable phonological system. Thus this type of treatment, introduced early enough, will prevent many of the phonological problems which can arise. This is based on the belief that articulation is the mechanical system of movement on which children build a sound system approximating to that of adults, by means of normal perceptual input, reliable self-monitoring and normally developing cognitive ability (Menn, 1980; Straight, 1980; Grunwell, 1985). Children achieve this sound system by hypothesizing how to equate the patterns which they are producing to match those in common use by adults (Ferguson, 1976). This involves, by repetition and monitoring, working out how to produce pronunciation patterns which sound both like those they hear in use around them and those by which they have already learned to comprehend heard language. In other words, normally developing children learn two systems of phonology. The initial system depends on cognitive and auditory factors and enables them to understand what others say to them. Simultaneously, they have to formulate, by cognition, memory and motor skills, how to produce their own pronunciation patterns for their own phonological system.

Clearly understanding this dichotomy between perception and production, between cognition and praxis, has created problems for some therapists working in the field. Contemporary teaching, from a baseline of linguistic knowledge, has clarified the situation for more recently qualified speech therapists. Those trained before linguistic studies were available are equipping themselves with current thinking by means of in-service courses. Unfortunately, more than acquaintance with current theories is required. Suitable clinical techniques have to be worked out to replace the more facile ones used before this stage of learning was reached. Earlier ideas of treatment by means of articulation drills are not applicable to language disorders such as delayed and/or deviant phonology. Neither do exercises for initial, medial and final placements, in isolation, help children whose difficulties lie in being unable to contrast and combine phonemes in order to employ the numerous permutations required to produce intelligible speech. A further barrier to clarification of this problem is the fact that there is disagreement in the terminology used in the English-speaking world with regard to the literature on the subject.

Phonological disorders is the term used in the UK. Many American writers still prefer the confusing term *functional articulation disorder*. The correct place for articulation drills and motor practice is in the area of speech and not in that of language, that is, in cases where there are either structural or neurological deviations from the normal, preventing children from articulating clearly. Phonology is a component of language.

Other craniofacial anomalies of various descriptions are being referred more often for speech therapy. The incidence of these abnormalities is small but three factors may increase referrals. Firstly, most infants are born in hospital and the medical profession has recognized that abnormal facial development may affect speech. Secondly, surgery has become more sophisticated and intervention for conditions such as hyperteliorism (a cranial anomaly in which the forehead, eyes and nasal bridge are abnormally stretched laterally in the middle third of the face) are more frequent. Realignment may improve the ability to articulate and also alter the resonance of the voice. Speech therapy may be required to redress the balance. Finally, educational circles at preschool levels are also inclined to refer children of this nature, although this is by no means generally practised.

To ascertain whether there are craniofacial, oropharyngeal neurophysiological or neuromuscular anomalies present, the speech therapist should *always* undertake an oral mechanism assessment.

An oral mechanism assessment should always be preceded by close observation of the general posture and movements of the child. For example:

1. Note the child's general posture and gait. Is there wide-based positioning of the feet?
2. Has the stage of using one foot after another on stairs been reached?
3. Does the child visually monitor her/his foot movements?
4. Has coordination developed fully in walking, running, jumping, skipping?
5. Have hand and finger movements matured?
6. Is there lateral awareness?
7. Does one hand appear to be dominant?
8. Have normal personal skills been acquired, e.g. washing, feeding, dressing?

9. Are basic educational skills developing, e.g. drawing, writing, reading?

All of this should be judged commensurately with normal age and developmental milestones. All deviations from normal should be noted. Now scrutinize the face for asymmetry, special feature characteristics such as deflected nasal septum, appropriate expressions during speech and any other anomalous signs. Then proceed to the oral examination proper (see Appendix C).

3

Developmental dysarthrias

Two major types of disorder constitute those which are described as being of neurological origin, these are dysarthria and dyspraxia. The former has been referred to in discussing the articulation disorder present in the speech of children with Down's syndrome, and will be dealt with first. Darley *et al.* (1975) indicate that:

> Dysarthria is a collective name for a group of related speech disorders that are due to disturbances in muscular control of the speech mechanism resulting from impairment of any of the basic motor processes involved in the execution of speech.
>
> (p. 2)

The basic motor processes referred to include breathing, phonation, resonance and articulation. In most cases of dysarthria each of these components is affected to a greater or lesser degree depending on the severity and site of the lesion. The major symptom is weakness of movement due to reduction of power and/or tone in the affected muscles. In addition, extraneous involuntary movements are frequently present, the nature of which is determined by the area of damage in the brain. Dysarthrias can be classified as follows:

1. *Type* Spastic
   Site Upper motor neurone (pyramidal tract)
   Speech disorder Rhythm disrupted; cannot direct or control breath due to inability to make velopharyngeal seal or to purse lips; poor laryngeal control interferes with phonation; difficulty

in protruding tongue, raising velum and controlling lip movement thus articulation is distorted; restrictions on velar movement affect resonance.

2. *Type* Athetoid
   Site Lower motor neurone
   Speech disorder Involuntary movements disrupt rhythm; dysphonia; better breath control than spastic; greater control of
   tongue and lips than spastic but involuntary writhing movements interfere, creating 'peristaltic' tongue movement; trial
   and error velar action may disrupt resonance.

3. *Type* Ataxic
   Site Cerebellum
   Speech disorder Over-compensatory movements affect direction and control of tongue, volume and pitch of voice and
   cause explosive, jerky articulation.

4. *Type* Hyperkinetic
   Site Extrapyramidal
   Speech disorder Exaggerated, uncontrolled flailing movements
   causing bizarre articulation and little control of phonation.

5. *Type* Hypokinetic
   Site Extrapyramidal
   Speech disorder Rigidity of muscles, reflexes diminished resulting in restricted range of movements; presence of tremor leads
   to festinant speech.

6. *Type* Mixed
   Site Multiple
   Speech disorder Combinations of above-named symptoms.

DYSPHAGIA

Dysphagia is the term given to difficulty in swallowing. This
condition results most frequently from either developmental
dysarthria which interferes with the acquisition of normal
muscular power and tone, or from acquired dysarthria following
disease or trauma which disturbs normal muscular power and
tone.

Several speech therapists have recently undertaken to work in
the field of dysphagia, arranging programmes for patients with
feeding difficulties caused by the dysarthrias. Since this is an area
of survival in both child and adult cases, clinicians have to consider

ethical, financial, insurance and professional aspects of the problem (The Dysphagia Series, in *Speech Therapy in Practice*, 1989).

Speech Therapy intervention for feeding should never be started until there has been comprehensive assessment and treatment by the medical team.

Langley's book, *Working with Swallowing Disorders* (1988), contains a comprehensive programme of treatment which includes emotional and safety factors as well as the considerations necessary for the physical management of such patients.

Feeding techniques (see Appendix D)

Several different aspects have to be considered before adopting a specific technique for feeding. For example, intraoral hypersensitivity may be present, in which case, desensitization will be required within the mouth. This may be achieved by teaching the carer to open the mouth in a gentle but firm grip and then to rub the gums, palate and alveolar ridge. Where a very strong bite reflex is present, it is advisable to carry out this routine using the back of a polythene spoon. The gag reflex can be reduced by gradually working from the front to the back of the tongue, using a polythene spoon once more, to apply pressure. This also helps to control tongue thrusting. After each part of these exercises close the child's jaw and encourage him to swallow.

When working with a child external tactile cueing may help to achieve controlled movement. Using the dominant hand, place the middle finger across the child's throat under the jaw with the forefinger along the jawbone to control lateral movement. Use the thumb to control lip closure. Tongue movements and swallowing are encouraged by gentle movement and pressure of the middle finger under the jaw and on the throat. Food should be presented at the front of a spoon placed at the midline of the mouth, and insistence should be placed on removing the food from the spoon with the upper lip. Care should be taken not to touch the teeth with the spoon as this may stimulate the bite reflex. To prevent excessive movement in the action of drinking, the rim of the cup should be placed between the lips and the jaw should be supported. Types of food used should be within and just above the child's capability as indicated by her/his level of maturation. Treharne (1980) suggests that the lips may be the key factor in a feeding management programme and, since they are so important, it may be possible to achieve good results by concentrating on them. She states that in normal development their function in feeding is to:

1. constrain the tongue during swallowing;
2. prevent escape of food;
3. form a seal to facilitate oral pressure changes.

In addition, the lips are the easiest organs to manipulate and desensitize of all the oral groups of muscles. It is, of course, essential to train all the adults concerned with a child in the system of feeding selected in order to maintain an attainable level of success for the child. Traumatic meal-time scenes are to be avoided at all costs, as serious long-term behaviour problems may result.

Occasionally the speech therapist may be asked to give an opinion on the feeding difficulties of infants of a few days or weeks in age. Experience has shown that such difficulties frequently are predictive of the presence of dysarthria, occurring as one of the constellation of symptoms present in one or other form of cerebral palsy. Medical staff are not specifically trained to recognize or to deal with infantile feeding problems and, because of this, time may often be lost in attempting either to improve present feeding techniques or in making alternative arrangements for feeding these infants, such as by tube feeding. This may account for 'failure to thrive' and should therefore be regarded as an important factor in paediatric care. For babies with inadequate palates, e.g. clefts, it is possible to provide an intraoral appliance to compensate for the anomaly and to enable them to perform adequate sucking and swallowing movements until surgical intervention can take place. The success of this type of appliance is dependent on the presence of an adequately working gag reflex, not always present in severe dysarthria (Selley and Boxall, 1986).

Hospitalized infants are regarded by some people as suffering from the deprivation of the mother/baby relationship afforded by breast feeding. In cases where it is possible for the baby to suck successfully, the mother may be able to remain in hospital with her child to meet this need. However, where muscular weakness is markedly present or where the infant is incubated this is not always successful or possible.

Richards (1980) discusses the social implications of infant feeding patterns. He feels that our infant feeding patterns are more a *result* of our social world than a *cause* of it as some people claim

(Erikson, 1964). It has been suggested that there is a correspondence in a society between the pattern of infant feeding and the style of adult relationships. In our society in which we meet numerous people in the course of our lives, most of our relationships are brief and distant. The only close relationships are between parents and children and between spouses. It has been argued that the intermittent patterning of infant feeding predisposes children towards this type of adult relationship and it is this argument with which Richards disagrees. He indicates the dangers of parents setting up a particular pattern of feeding in the expectation that it will produce a baby with a certain kind of temperament. Feeding therapy has been carefully described by several workers including speech therapists (Treharne, 1980; Warner, 1981).

Talbot (1988), working with premature babies in London, notes, among other aspects:

1. how long it takes to complete a feed;
2. what difficulties are encountered by staff and parents in feeding;
3. how easily sucking is elicited, its rhythm, strength and speed;
4. adequacy of the lip seal;
5. normalcy of tongue movements – abnormal postures involve retraction or protrusion;
6. coughing and choking;
7. gagging – present, absent or hypersensitive.

With this and further information she is then able to plan management which in turn can be undertaken by nursing staff and parents.

MOTOR SCHEMAS

It is appropriate at this stage to look briefly at a schema theory applied to speech development. There are several proponents of such theories but the one which appears to be most applicable is that of Schmidt (1975a, b, 1976) which was later applied to speech by Kent (1982). Possibly the greatest strength of Schmidt's work is its emphasis on the *learning*, rather than simply the *performance*, of a motor skill. Schema theory is based on two separate states of memory. *Recall memory*, which generates commands for movement to the muscles, and *recognition memory* which, in turn, evaluates the response-produced feedback for monitoring purposes.

It is also necessary to assume that the Central Nervous System (CNS) forms 'generalized' motor programmes that consist of all the details of the motor commands required to carry out a movement. The two different types of memory perform different roles. Rapid movements are completely under the control of recall memory, recognition memory only being activated to register any errors by comparing expected sensory consequences with actual sensory consequences, on the completion of the act. Slow movements allow ongoing adjustments for errors and so both recall and recognition memories will be in use. Thus the schema derives from the relationship between experience of initial conditions, past results and response programmes – the recall schema – and of initial conditions, sensory consequences and actual results – the recognition schema. Such schemata allow the speaker to predict outcomes, to refine actions on the basis of past errors (i.e. to learn) and to perform skilfully even when a new motor programme is required. Kent (1982) suggests that the schema is a useful abstraction describing the motor control of speech in the same way that the phoneme is a useful abstraction in phonology. Further research is required to refine this theory but at present it serves a useful role in going some way to explain how an articulatory gesture can be used to mediate changes in meaning, e.g. /pan/ to /nap/, how gesture can change from being effortful to becoming automatic and why there are so many possible routes by which children become skilled speakers.

Kent believes that dysarthric children have difficulty in establishing the basic schema for speech. This, he suggests is due to impairments in motor performance and deficits in the monitoring and integration of sensory feedback. The schema theory supports the successful therapeutic approaches already discussed, e.g. strong breath support for speech, slowed rate of utterance, syllabic production and overarticulation. The ensuing problems of inability to learn such schema are therefore serious. If a motor programme is formulated only by selection and use of previously learned motor commands, and since new speech sounds cannot apparently be learned by any other means but from drawing on previously experienced and internalized memories, it would appear that this theory indicates that there can be no improvement for children with moderate or severe degrees of dysarthria.

MATURATION

It appears more and more significant to the writer, from research findings to be described later (p. 52), and from empirical clinical results, that insufficient consideration is paid to maturation. Children born with a disability which has dysarthria as one of its symptoms frequently have multiple defects such as visual, auditory and kinaesthetic deficits. They also appear to have a decelerated rate of maturation. In other words, they take appreciably longer to acquire some skills than their undamaged contemporaries. This is of vital importance to professionals working with such children and to the nature of counselling which is given to parents and carers. It seems likely that there will be a residual amount of difficulty depending on the severity of the initial damage or dysfunction after the child has reached maximum maturity, but that the retarded acquisition of maturity in itself will account for some of the early difficulties experienced.

When considering the development of language, Lenneberg (1967) suggested that human beings reached their potential for language learning in their adolescent teenage period. He said that this meant that, for example, people with Down's syndrome (DS) stopped developing language at approximately 14 years old and that they would continue to use the delayed language level that they had reached by that time. There is evidence now that this is not the case. Cunningham (1982) suggests that in the more able person with Down's syndrome, mental growth, which includes language, can continue into at least the late thirties.

If the experience of people with disabilities resembles that of the normal population this is an underestimate in the case of those healthy but handicapped people. Experience indicates that learning continues throughout the whole of life and that this will be the case in healthy, normal and disabled people. However, the rate, as well as the depth, of learning will depend on the overall capabilities of each individual. Time must be given when dealing with the disabled to exploit those capabilities beyond the limit which may be used with supposedly normal adults.

Cerebral palsy

In conditions resulting in irreversible brain damage such as cerebral palsy, maturation is one of the two factors which are not always sufficiently acknowledged. The other factor is degree of severity. On numerous occasions parents have been told that their child will never walk, talk or in any way develop in a near-normal way. Frequently those predictions have been proved wrong. It appears that in many cases this is due to concentrated physical exercises. The submission being made here is that there has to be a possible attainable level for each individual and that maturation plays a large part in determining that level. Where children appear to be unable to improve, it seems likely that there is such severe damage that improvement cannot occur, or that persistent immaturity prevents it. In some cases both factors are present.

There is no doubt that, for many children, it is necessary to start the process for change in a passive manner. That is, the actions to be aimed for may require an external agent to demonstrate them to initiate the movements as the child will have no access to memorized sensory feedback loops from which to base stimulation of the groups of muscles involved. Brain damage has long lasting and serious effects on child development. Lack of, or disordered, mobility prevents the child from going through the endless movements which normally start pre-natally and which build up the sensory feedback on which all movement is based. Practice of gross and fine motor activity is required in almost all parts of the body to facilitate development. Research has provided us with very little information in this area so far. Might it not be possible that infants' apparently endless experiments with movement stimulate the necessary myelination to establish locomotion, manual dexterity, eye-movements and the movements of articulation? Thus, although children with cerebral palsy will not achieve smoothness and speed of movement to a normal degree there is a level to which most can aspire.

In addition to the awareness that children with cerebral palsy need help in learning how to move, parents of such children have two factors with which to contend. These are acceptance and understanding of the situation. Little or no help is given on either aspect, although a great deal of information is now known both about the power of discussion with people in a similar situation and about the whys, the wherefores and the 'how to cope with' such children. Too many parents are left to work things out for themselves from total ignorance of the working of the human brain. The result is that too many children are taken for help at too late a stage in their maturational development and after they have missed out on too many critical periods of learning. This situation may improve as people are no longer satisfied with being left in a state of ignorance about crucial aspects of the human condition. Also, medical workers are becoming aware of the need to inform patients and relatives of conditions and situations which have to be coped with on both short- and long-term bases, e.g. use of signing for communication in absence of speech.

Cerebral palsy is defined as a disorder of posture, movement and tone due to a lesion or maldevelopment of the immature brain (McKinlay, personal communication). There is an incidence of about 2:1000 live births. Males are more commonly affected, about 55%. About 50% of all people with cerebral palsy are of normal intelligence, about 6% are of superior intelligence, roughly 25% present with moderate learning disability and the remaining 20% with severe learning disability. Several associated problems can be found in children with cerebral palsy, such as epilepsy and difficulties with sight and hearing, but the greatest of the problems are those of movement. Cerebral palsy takes several forms, each determined by the site of lesion. The dysarthrias resulting also vary according to the part of the cerebrum or cerebellum affected. A paediatric neurologist should be able to diagnose whether the state is present and predict which form it is likely to take from about 4–6 months of age, but it may be later before the degree of severity can be determined.

Most common types of cerebral palsy are as follows:

1. Spastic (about 65%) increase in tone in affected limbs and bulbar muscles;
2. Athetoid (5 to 10%) involuntary movement at rest increased on voluntary exertion, tongue affected;
3. Rigid (5 to 10%) increase in tone throughout full range of movement;
4. Ataxic (5%) disturbed equilibrium, intention tremor;
5. Mixed (10%) combined features of above.

Physiotherapy constitutes the greater part of treatment in cerebral palsy. In the early stages, the speech therapist may be asked to help with feeding. Parent counselling in the use of normal language and encouragement in conversational interchange is vital as children with cerebral palsy, more than most, need every form of practice. The dysarthrias, which differ according to the site of lesion, would be managed as in all dysarthrias. Alternative or agumentative forms of communication, e.g. computers, light readers, Cannon communicators, should be used where necessary.

Supra-bulbar palsy

A comparatively rare developmental defect of the motor tract is supra-bulbar palsy which affects the tenth and twelfth cranial nerves, the vagus (X) and hypoglossal (XII). This is a specific defect in which there are usually no other associated neurological abnormalities present. Symptoms present as follows (Worster-Drought, 1974):

1. velum most frequently affected; when mild, elevation is restricted and movements are slow; when severe, complete paralysis results. Nasal escape will be present in relation to the degree of severity;
2. tongue will prove difficult to elevate;
3. lips will only be affected in severest cases when protrusion may be impossible;
4. pharyngeal and/or laryngeal muscles are seldom involved.

MANAGEMENT

Assessment

Although it is necessary to assess in all types of speech/language disorders, the process of assessment for dysarthrias is particularly important as the type of dysarthria is determined according to the site of lesion in the brain. Symptomatology varies according to the type and, in turn, determines management (p. 37).

The two foremost tests in the UK are The Frenchay Dysarthria Assessment (FDA) (Enderby, 1983) and Robertson's Dysarthria Profile (RDP) (Robertson, 1982). The latter is essentially a descriptive assessment designed to identify the client's motor problems regardless of the neurological aetiology. Thus, no attempt is made to discriminate between different types of dysarthria. However, experience in its use shows that this profile lends itself to the planning of appropriate clinical management. Alternatively, the FDA enables clinicians to differentiate between the main types of dysarthrias. In 1984, Enderby and Rowarth published microcomputer software associated with the FDA which produces a precise differential diagnosis of each of the five major groups of dysarthrias based on the data resulting from the administration of the FDA. Consensus from clinicians indicates that the ability to make such a differential diagnosis is the strongest feature of the FDA, although claims are made in the manual that it is readily applicable to therapy.

As they have much experience in listening to 'dysarthric speech' and frequently know what the client's response is likely to be, clinicians are inclined to rate intelligibility higher than it actually is. In the RDP this has been considered and not only the speech therapist, but also family and friends of the client are asked to assess intelligibility. Thus, a more realistic assessment of the client's speech will result.

Instrumentation has also been widely used in the assessment of the dysarthrias. For example, Kent and Netsell (1975) and Kent (1982) have produced spectrographic studies which illustrate the usefulness of this technique, particularly when applied to dysarthrias.

Treatment

Dworkin (1984) considers that there are four important clinical principles:

1. type of dysarthria and its neuromuscular and speech signs must be identified;
2. aetiology and medical diagnosis may dictate nature and timing of treatments;
3. prognosis is dependent on severity, aetiology and success of medical intervention;
4. short- and long-term objectives are usually more realistic than the treatment plan which focuses on restoring normal motor skills and speech proficiency.

Numerous approaches are used by different clinicians, most include the following in some form or other:

1. resistance to passive movement;
2. proprioceptive neuromuscular facilitation, including icing, brushing and stroking;

3. increase of range of movement;
4. timing, rhythmic and resonance exercises;
5. specific labial, lingual, palatal, nasal/oral awareness, velo-pharyngeal and laryngeal exercises;
6. articulation training and practice leading to use of words, phrases and sentences;
7. appropriate prosodic use.

Environmental factors

A further crucial element in the ability of disabled children, such as those with dysarthria, to develop near-normal skills depends on the nature of their earliest environmental experiences. There is virtually no attempt to educate or even familiarize future parents with any knowledge of rearing children. In a few schools, parentcraft discussions do take place. Unfortunately, neither the specific consideration of the development of language nor the possibility of having to cope with a handicapped child are often considered. The importance of mother-child bonding has been relatively widely studied, but rarely is there any mention of the possibility of the birth of a handicapped child. In such an eventuality some parents need help and support to accept the situation before they can begin to relate closely to the child. Quantities of tender, loving care may be available in such situations, but the mother may experience great difficulty in accepting the need to set up a normal mother-child dyad for the acquisition of language by the child. And the problem is not entirely that of the mother.

In her paper, Jones (1975) compared six mother-normal infant dyads with six mother-Down's syndrome infant dyads matched for mental age (8–19 months). Her six major categories were as follows:

1. direction of mother's eye-gaze;
2. non-vocal activity of mother;
3. vocal activity of mother;
4. direction of child's eye-gaze;
5. non-vocal activity of child;
6. vocal activity of child.

Jones recorded no difference of frequency of participation in inter-actions by Down's syndrome children, normal children and their respective mothers. Despite no significant differences in overall frequency of eye-contact for the two groups, the normal children used much more referential looking than the Down's syndrome children. There were no differences in the vocalizations produced by both groups but the Down's syndrome children left very little space between their utterances, making it very difficult for their mothers to establish a dialogue. The Down's syndrome children often vocalized at the same time as their mothers, whereas the normal children structured their utterances in such a way as to facilitate a dialogue. In addition, the mothers of the Down's syndrome children initiated more interactive sequences with their children whereas the mothers of normal children structured their interactions in response to cues from their children. Jones concluded that although the Down's syndrome children provided sufficient cues to maintain a comparable rate of interaction with their mothers, the quality of their interaction was somewhat different.

In a larger study, Rondal (1978) considered the language of 21 Down's syndrome children, 21 normal children and their respective mothers in a free-play situation in their homes for two 30 min sessions. The children were matched on the basis of the mean length of utterances (MLU) used by the children. This is an unusual and unique matching basis. It assumes that mothers simplify their speech to their children on the basis of the language ability of the children rather than on chronological or mental age. Results revealed that the two groups differed in only two aspects, the type-token ratio and the number of imitated utterances. The Down's syndrome children used many more inappropriate verbalizations and imitated less than the normal children. This indicates that the handicapped child participates less in structuring interactions than the normal child.

Beveridge and Lloyd (1977) claim that mothers are the primary mediators of the meanings of children's first messages. They suggest that the child develops in an ever increasing close-knit participation with his/her mother in understanding the world, and that their response to each other is so sensitive as to make them share a joint construct. In other words 's/he sees what she sees what s/he sees'. This explains why the wider language community relies so heavily on linguistic cues and less so on extra-linguistic cues. These writers also suggest that mothers of handicapped children have had more interpretative practice with their children's communications so may therefore better understand ambiguous utterances which others fail to interpret. However, another factor has to be considered at this point. Not infrequently, mothers fail to provide this participative interchange so necessary for the development of normal language. The two most common reasons for this failure are firstly, that the mother is unaware of her role in the interaction, and/or secondly, that she herself has a linguistic or communicative problem. There continue to be mothers who, when asked to present their offspring for a speech therapy assessment, claim that they do not speak to them because the child is too young to reply. Such mothers need careful counselling and help to assume the role of modeller and teacher. In fact, speech therapists are presently aiming to assist mothers to be their own therapists and to enable them to guide their infants and toddlers through the beginning stages of language development in these circumstances when it appears that the baby is behind in acquiring the expected skills (Weistuch and Byers Brown, 1987).

Other domestic factors may also be operating against some children learning language. It is a common occurrence for children to be brought up in one-parent families. Frequently this situation is completely successful and such children seem to suffer no ill effects. There is a percentage, however, that lose out in these circumstances from anxiety of several types, possibly financial, emotional, or illness-created. Another problem arising, or perhaps of only recent recognition, is the increase in child abuse. It must also be admitted that this often occurs within the family. Where there is fear in a familiar situation there is a threat to learning, and skills are not always acquired within the expected time limits. Further, in older children, this situation may provoke different speech difficulties such as selective mutism, in which a child elects not to use the language at his/her disposal in situations of threat and/or exposure (p. 96).

4

Developmental articulatory dyspraxia

This chapter is concerned with the second aspect of neurological impairments which affect the normal development of speech in children.

Dyspraxia is the term used to denote an inability to perform voluntarily, specific motor actions, on command or demonstration, consistently on all occasions, in the absence of any major neurophysiological or neuromuscular disability (Milloy, 1985). The particular dyspraxia being considered is *developmental articulatory dyspraxia* (DAD). 'Developmental' indicates that the condition occurs in developing children. The term 'articulatory' minimizes confusion in the consideration of the speech production element of the problem and 'dyspraxia' represents a partial rather than a total disturbance of praxis. Several other terms are used to denote this condition. That commonly employed in the USA is developmental apraxia of speech. Children may be born with one or several of all the various types of developmental dyspraxia, for example, limb, ideomotor, ideational, oral, constructional. It is important to determine whether a child suspected of having DAD has any other forms of dyspraxia as their presence may influence management of DAD. The nature of DAD seems to result from a *motor planning inadequacy*.

Darley *et al.* (1975) describe motor planning or programming as resulting from the action of the motor speech programmer (MSP). They speculate that the MSP may be driven by three possible forces. Firstly, they feel that for most language operations the MSP is driven and directed by the central language processor (CLP), which they describe as having as one of its functions the selection of words and sequences of words which transform meaningful internal content into language for externalization.

After the selection, the CLP converts the word sequences into a neural code of directions for the MSP which, in turn, initiates motor planning or programming. Darley *et al.* maintain that this process involves

> the selective activation of some hundred muscles important to speech at the proper time, in the proper order, and for the correct duration to produce the desired speech sounds in the desired sequence. If the figure of 14 is taken as a reasonable rate of phoneme production per second, and if the average speech muscle comprises 100 motor units, the production of speech must require 140 000 neuromuscular events per second. This implies that the formation of speech sounds is the result of pre-programmed chains of neural output.
>
> (p. 258)

Hogg and Moss (1983) describe motor programming as:

> the integration of a set of previously independent but well-learned individual movements into a sequence which, once consolidated, can be adapted easily to meet the environmental constraints of the task.

Darley *et al.* (1975) contend, however, that:

> clinical evidence indicates that it is possible to have impairment of motor speech (apraxia of speech) with little or no impairment of the functions of language.

Consider this in the light of the work of Stark (1980) who indicated that normally developing children, after several months of random and then meaningful babbling, appear to automatize their articulatory skills, that is, motor skills for articulation become automatic before a child's first birthday. Milloy (1985) found that children with moderate and severe degrees of DAD were reported by their parents as *not having babbled*, that is, they had not become skilled in the selection and manipulation of those muscles required for the use of correct and automatic articulation. This omission in their developmental progress may account for the dyspraxic habit which prevents them producing intelligible speech.

DAD v. IAP

Milloy devised a procedure to identify the presence of DAD which was found to be successful in revealing the presence of DAD after three, or preferably five, applications at six-monthly intervals (Milloy Assessment of Praxis, MAP). However, an unexpected revelation issued from the test results produced after such intervals. Not only was it possible to identify DAD, but also a second condition was found in some cases. The results of some of the children varied minimally from administration to administration, while the results of the majority who started out also apparently presenting with DAD were discovered to be showing improvement over the periods of testing. It was then possible to claim that those children had a condition which was resolving with maturation.

This condition was termed *immature articulatory praxis* (IAP). In the case of children with IAP it appears that their later maturation means later automatization of their articulatory skills. When questioned, parents of the IAP children remembered that there had been some, but not a great deal of babbling occurring during their earliest months. Simultaneously, these children who were immature in their articulatory development apparently reached a level of autonomy for oral praxis preceding the establishment of articulatory praxis which is missing in the skills' ability of children with DAD.

Milloy's study (1985), although dealing with a relatively small number of children with DAD, found that all of them had oral dyspraxia contrary to the claims made by other workers (Rosenbek, 1980; Guyette and Diedrich, 1981). The former not only suggests that oral dyspraxia indicates neuromotor involvement of the speech mechanism but that it *may* accompany both DAD and stuttering. (Oral dyspraxia is present when the individual is unable to copy voluntary movements of the oral organs, e.g. tongue, lips, on command or demonstration in the absence of attempts to articulate.) It seems likely that oral dyspraxia *always* accompanies DAD and *occasionally* accompanies IAP. According to Guyette and Diedrich (1981), 'oral and articulatory dyspraxia do not necessarily co-exist'. This may be a further means of differentiating between DAD and IAP. It certainly seems feasible that those children with a motor programming dysfunction will exhibit it in the oral as well as the articulatory dimensions of motor activity, while those whose problem is one of maturity will use movements which manifest patchy, or incomplete ability. As indicated, careful assessment to determine the presence of either DAD or IAP is the first essential in dealing with those children.

Planning management for both conditions will be similar depending on the degree of severity of the condition to be treated (Milloy and Morgan-Barry, 1990). In each case it is extremely difficult to determine degrees of severity due to the presence of so many idiosyncratic variables in the speech of each individual. Some children will go through life presenting with a mild degree of difficulty which will resist treatment and never change and which should be regarded as being a mild form of DAD. Similarly, moderate or severe degrees of either DAD or IAP will occur in certain cases. A further point to consider in planning treatment for both types of difficulty is the presence of other accompanying dyspraxic or immature factors.

As already stated, such dyspraxic tendencies may affect movements of the limbs, the digits, the eyes and the initiation and execution of more complex groups of movements, such as those required for writing. In the most severe cases clinicians' awareness of the presence of one or some of those types of dyspraxia is necessary before embarking on, for example, an alternative communicative system such as signing. Similarly, in the case of immaturity, assessment of cognitive and other related abilities should be made to ensure that the programme of treatment is within the capabilities of the child. In both cases, a 'whole-person' approach should be contemplated, which will be instrumental in availing the child of maximum improvement. Since there are many similarities in the conditions at the initial stages, management will also be the same.

Milloy (1985) alluded to two further important issues resulting from the investigation to identify the presence of DAD: 1) DAD is of rare occurrence; 2) DAD is a natural basis for a phonological disorder.

An experiment was designed which assessed the motor skills of four groups of children:

10 preschool children	: age range 3;0–4;0
10 schoolchildren	: age range 6;0–8;0
10 children with moderate learning difficulties (MLD)	: age range 6;0–9;0

10 children with severe language   : age range 6;0–9;0
impairments (LI)

Each child was assessed over a period of 12 months on three occasions on the MAP and the Edinburgh Articulation Test (EAT) (Anthony *et al.*, 1971). Results showed that of the total of 40 children, six had DAD. Sixteen had IAP to a greater or a lesser degree including all the children with MLD, the four remaining children with LI and two of the preschool children. Eighteen children had normal motor skill ability for articulation. Claims could thus be made that DAD is of rare occurrence. The children presenting with it had been withdrawn from normal school on the grounds that their language/speech impairment interfered with their ability to cope with mainstream schooling. None of the children in the other three groups had DAD. Continued testing has shown that all the children with IAP have eventually acquired articulatory praxis. (On further investigation it was acknowledged that children with DAD are also liable to immaturity which eventually disappears with maturation.) The children with DAD, five of whom were later found also to have IAP which has since been resolved, continue to have a residual core of DAD which is resistant to either treatment or to maturation (Milloy and Summers, 1990).

The speech samples elicited at the final time of testing within the experiment were analysed on the Phonological Assessment of Child Speech (PACS) (Grunwell, 1985). Results produced a further revelation with clinical implications. Those children with DAD evidenced irrefutable signs of phonological disorder. The phonological involvement corresponded in severity with that of DAD. Those children with the most severe DAD used restricted pronunciation patterns, for example, 'favourite articulations' as described by Ingram (1979). Phonotactic possibilities were greatly reduced in the speech of those children, with only consonant-vowel (CV), vowel-consonant (VC) and occasional consonant-vowel-consonant (CVC) occurring. Thus it can be claimed that DAD acted as the natural basis for a phonological disorder (Harris and Cottam, 1985). Alternatively, children with IAP were all evincing language, including phonological, delay.

Spatial/temporal aspects

Spatial and temporal awareness and perceptual and productive skills should be checked simultaneously and the child enabled to improve on all those areas. Use of a visual perceptive programme may facilitate this (Frostig and Horne, 1966). Music and rhythm are known to be centred in the right hemisphere and language primarily in the left. There is therefore associated integration between the appreciation of time such as motor rhythms and cognitive intention and interpretation. Many children with DAD and IAP have considerable timing difficulties. Some appear to be in the area of processing information, but it may well be that the real problem lies with the time it takes to organize and plan the motor aspects of the response. Motor memories (p. 46) may be unreliable.

It seems unlikely that children will be able to react to linguistic rules unless they can identify themselves in time and space. Children with DAD appear to have specific problems in these areas and are frequently unable to operate normally in all circumstances.

Deixis

This is the use of spatial, temporal and interpersonal features of linguistic and non-linguistic context to provide joint reference (Lee, 1979). It is often a closed book to such children. It is of particular interest to consider the relationship between deixis, which is derived from the Greek word for 'pointing', and ideomotor dyspraxia, which, in one form, is a failure to indicate by pointing. Children with DAD may appear confused in the use of several deictic categories, particularly:

1. personal pronouns, e.g. I, you, she, mine, yours, hers;
2. impersonal pronouns, e.g. this, that, these, those;
3. adverbs, e.g. here, there, now, then, left, right;
4. prepositions, e.g. up, down; inside, outside; in, on.

All these linguistic forms are reliant on the clear appreciation of oneself in space and time. It is sometimes necessary to teach children how to handle these concepts which they do not develop automatically (Appendix B).

55

Crystal (1981b) describes a situation of the opposite type in which a child relies considerably on deictic expression and thus produces a semantically 'empty' language (pp. 121–125). It is much more common for children, especially those with moderate learning difficulties, to have problems appreciating deictic requirements. Many of those children are found to have IAP, a degree of clumsiness of movement and a 'fuzzy' concept of their personal identities.

Pursuing the relevance of appreciation of deixis and its categories, which are dependent on the knowledge of spatial relationships between one object and another, Bryant (1980), when discussing occupational therapy, emphasizes the need to work on this ability when undertaking body image training. She points out that the child may need to experience these positions for her/himself first before being able to relate them to outside her/himself.

Interpersonal and intrapersonal awareness

There are two levels at which children experience space and time, the intrapersonal and the interpersonal. While the majority of children with both DAD and IAP can identify facial and limbic features with ease, they frequently have difficulty with more complex parts of their bodies, e.g. the back of the left knee, the middle of the forehead. This indicates an uncertainty within the child about his/her own personal topography, without which general spatial awareness becomes difficult (intrapersonal). Likewise, whilst able to identify common objects like doors, windows, chairs, etc. by pointing, some children find specific spatial identification more difficult, e.g. pointing to the chair *behind* the table, the plant *outside* the window (interpersonal/figure-background).

It is sometimes necessary to take the child through the motions of identifying spatial relationships, e.g. pointing to the chair behind the table then moving towards it, touching it, naming it, if possible, and perhaps, in situations of great difficulty, drawing it in line form in relation to the table. It can be a waste of time to expect some children to proceed to more complex spatial situations until this initial stage has been firmly established. It is always important to remember that such children have motor memory deficits and that these may affect movements other than those of articulation. A useful exercise is to ask the child to lie on a large sheet of paper on the floor while his/her outline is drawn. S/he is then able to appreciate him/herself by studying, discussing, drawing over, standing upright her/his lifesize representation.

In addition to appreciating position, children need to recognize dimensions such as different sizes, amounts and shapes, especially in fine variations. It is always profitable to explore these aspects in concrete forms before resorting to the use of symbolic representations; that is, make sure that the child can identify by sight, hearing, feel, touch and smell all the properties of body schemata, clothing, common household objects such as toiletries, foodstuffs, cleaning agents and so on, before expecting him/her to recognize aspects of pictures and other symbols.

Experts in other areas consider the development of autonomy in the appreciation of space and proportion in different contexts. For example, Quin and Macauslan (1986) state that:

> the young child gets his first ideas of space and proportion by moving in space. The more chairs he crawls under, the more sofas he climbs over the better.
>
> (p. 277)

They feel that the more experience the child has of such things as unpacking shopping, moving and regrouping spoons, helping with baking, observing dials on gadgets, etc. the quicker s/he will learn number, i.e. numeracy and eventually reading. Talking with the child about all these familiar subjects which rely on spatial, and also temporal, knowledge will lay foundations for the understanding of the basic educational skills expected of the normal school beginner.

It is obvious that children with motor programming difficulties will take longer to sort out the levels of understanding which their normally developing peers appear to learn so easily. With DAD and IAP children there is wide variability and variation in the range of difficulties.

Re-assessment of 'clumsy' children has been made recently. Henderson (1987) alludes to the fact that for some children there seems to be no motor activity which they can manage with ease, while others appear to have more specific problems focused perhaps on cutting with scissors, using a knife and fork, learning to form letters for writing or using speech which lacks clarity and fluency. He lists traditional assessments under three headings:

57

1. 'descriptive' tests
2. 'diagnostic' tests
3. 'neurodevelopmental' test batteries.

In the first category he includes the Test of Motor Impairment (Stott *et al*., 1984) and points out that under the age of four no clear distinction tends to be drawn between tests of motor competence and tests of cognitive competence, so he refers to the Bayley Scales (1969) and the Griffiths Test (1954). Among 'diagnostic' tests Henderson mentions the Developmental Test of Visual Perception (Frostig and Horne, 1966), the Purdue Perceptual-Motor Survey (Roach and Kephart, 1966) and the Southern California Sensory Integration Tests (Ayres, 1972).

To this point the discussion has been at the level of motor planning and the ensuing motor control. This can become somewhat confusing unless the close relationship between sensory and motor development is remembered and it is understood that the sensory factors are implicit in all discussions of motor deficits. The three last-mentioned tests take this into account. 'Diagnostic' tests purport to measure such aspects as 'body image' and 'tactile defensiveness'. Although it is acknowledged that among children described as 'clumsy' a very small proportion will be suffering from an identifiable neurological condition, it is common paediatric practice to carry out a full neurological assessment. Hall (1983) suggested the following definition of a 'neurodevelopmental' test:

> a clinical examination – designed to supplement the classical
> neurological examination in order to reveal subtle deficiencies
> in neurological function and whose interpretation is age-
> dependent.

This definition is attractive for two reasons. It describes dysfunction, not damage, that is, it allows for the inconsistency factor which so frequently accompanies dyspraxia. Furthermore, it precludes maturational influences. However, all of these assessments are of too general a nature and fail to describe the problem, diagnose the condition or provide directives for practical guidance in helping children with such difficulties.

Henderson points out that the qualitative observation checklists added to the 'normative' record forms provided by the Test of Motor Impairment (Stott *et al*., 1984) are intended to describe the common faults characteristic of poor performers. This approach is also the one adopted by Milloy (1985) in designing MAP. Observations are made and recorded of how each item is performed by each child and a fine descriptive system of the production patterns produced by each child is employed to indicate idiosyncratic individual performances. Evidence is thus available of the quantification and the qualitative factors of the spatial properties of the articulatory mechanisms and their component parts as they change over time.

Checks should also be made of feeding techniques. Experience to date indicates that there are problems in this area only when dyspraxia co-exists with dysarthria.

Treatment proceeds towards, where possible, the acquisition of reliable consistent production by means of visual, proprioceptive and tactile feedback loop systems. The ideal position for this section of management is for clinician and client to sit side by side facing a large mirror in which each can monitor his/her own and the other's attempts to achieve target placements. It must be ascertained that left-right awareness is fully established. This left-right awareness will have been covered in the preliminary exercises and assessments made to determine treatment readiness (Frostig and Horne, 1966). Before each session, using a mirror, recapitulate for the child the positions, movements and functions of the oral and facial features. Begin with the visible movements of the lips: openness, closure, protrusion and retraction without phonation. Now introduce /p/,/b/ and /m/. Remind the child of voicing by demonstration and imitation. Contrast /p/ and /b/ for this purpose. Remind the child of the nasal/oral contrast using /b/ and /m/.

Dean and Howell (1986) (Howell and Dean, 1987) in their clinical approach – Metaphon – provide a useful means of teaching children how to become aware of contrasting features independently of speech production. Children with moderate to severe IAP and/or phonological disorders may learn contrasts and feature differences more successfully by using Metaphon than by initial direct methods. The absence of repeated failure is surely the most important influence in this approach. The client will usually have had personal, and possibly painful, experience of failure and will need to be motivated to overcome frustration as well as to improve performance. This demands a positive approach by the clinician. Success is only possible in short, well-planned bursts of absolutely appropriate treatment initially. However, normalcy must be ensured. Treatment has been observed during which contrived productions are accepted. The tendency to over-emphasize can detract from acceptable use of the sounds of the language and unnatural articulation may result. It is always necessary to retain the interacting sounds of English which result from constant changes in juxtapositions and which are not achieved by isolated sound practice. Also, possibly the greatest teaching aid is meaningfulness, and no reduction of this should be made over any but the shortest of practice periods.

Inevitably failures will occur in the normal course of therapy sessions, but it is crucial that the first stages make it possible for the child to succeed to some extent. To achieve this success very small expectations should be the immediate aim. Also, the parents, teachers and others concerned with the child should be clearly instructed in the vital first steps to enable them to maintain the ground gained. Possibly the suggested visible lip movements and contrasts will be sufficient for the child to cope with at the first meeting. Experience has shown that frequently too much is both aimed for and tried in the early stages of management. More than any other consideration, this can be instrumental in losing the child's confidence and therefore in preventing any early signs of either improvement or enthusiasm.

The child's general abilities should be investigated at the initial interview. By planning a simple ball game it should be possible to determine how well the child can stand, walk, run and jump, while, at the same time checking on her/his ability to catch, kick and generally control a ball. Again, clinical observation has shown that often too little time is given to this kind of activity to ascertain the child's real ability. This may result from a feeling that this type of activity is not within the remit of the speech therapist. On the contrary, particularly in cases of motor disability, it is essential to discover the whole-person praxis.

Articulation is simply one aspect of a human being's motor skills. All skills interact with each other and reflect each other in their performance. Further, the inclusion of a more general, energetic activity will renew the client's motivation and refresh his/her body and mind to return to less interesting, but necessary, specific exercises. A child suspected of having DAD/IAP is often older than would be desired before the correct diagnosis is made. This calls for more imagination in the programme of management. Reading, writing and mathematics may all be affected as a result of the presence of DAD or IAP. These are all language-linked subjects and may have to be included in the work done with the speech therapist. The class teacher should be contacted and an attempt made to work together, each contributing his/her specific expertise to formulate the best means of devising a learning approach for the child to use. The spatial, temporal, motor and general learning abilities of the child should form the baseline for treatment.

Management

After testing for spatial/temporal awareness and basic vocal tract development, treatment should begin with assessment of the basic skills of articulation, breathing, phonating, resonating and articulating, as already discussed.

ARTICULATION

After establishing lip movements, or, in the case of moderate-severe DAD identifying lip dyspraxia, proceed to tongue movements. Sitting side-by-side in front of a mirror, experiment and explore all the possible positions of the tongue and test for the child's ability to copy movements on command and by demonstration. The criteria for a controlled tongue in the protruded position are:

1. the ability to protrude tongue in isolation with no support from lower teeth or lip or other means;
2. the ability to hold tongue reasonably still in above position;
3. the ability to keep tongue in the mid-line in this position;
4. turn tongue up to touch nose;
5. turn tongue down to touch chin;
6. move tip of tongue from one corner of the mouth to the other several times, as quickly as possible;
7. move tip of tongue over total surface of the lips several times.

Proceed to jaw movements:

1. open the mouth wide, then close;
2. wiggle the jaw from side to side;
3. simulate chewing movements.

To test breath direction and control:

1. keep mouth closed, fill cheeks with air then expel air by punching cheeks and causing an explosive emission of air;
2. whistle (few, if any, children with DAD/IAP can whistle).

This assessment checks for the presence of *oral* dyspraxia only.

To assess for tongue involvement in *articulatory* dyspraxia it is necessary to test the behaviour of the tongue during articulation. The tongue-tip movements are seen in /t/, /d/ and /n/. The back-of-tongue movements are involved in producing /k/, /g/ and /ŋ/. Unfortunately, these cannot be so easily observed, if at all. However, the expert ear soon becomes tuned to the segments being produced by children with 'backing' difficulties.

As well as the clarity and precision of production of all these segments, the clinician should also be listening for examples of inconsistency and sequencing problems. These can be detected when several attempts are made with each production, e.g. /t,t,t/ /d,d,d/.

To test the ability to succeed in the production of these segments at greater depth, it is useful, after the initial separate practice of each, to produce them in groups, e.g.

/p,t,k/; /p,t,k/; /p,t,k/
/b,d,g/; /b,d,g/; /b,d,g/.

In addition to listening and watching, the child should be encouraged to feel what happens as he/she produces the different movements. To access the proprioceptive level for the child, it may be necessary to use pressure to stimulate feeling. The child with DAD, and to a lesser extent, the child with IAP have difficulty in establishing sensory feedback loop systems due to the unreliability of their motor movements for articulation, created by the defect in motor planning. Exaggeration of the pressure of, for example, the tip of the tongue on the centre of the alveolar ridge may stimulate sufficient feeling for the child to create a memorable sensation which may be recalled the next time the sound has to be produced.

After a lengthy period during which a child has had inconsistent and failing experiences in producing segments for articulation, a considerable amount of time will be required to eradicate erroneous methods, and replace them with correct ones.

Phonation

Voice onset is frequently unreliable in DAD and should be consciously practised. Thibodeau and Sussman (1979) and Daniloff *et al.* (1981) agreed on results of investigations into voice onset time (VOT) recorded by groups of normal and misarticulating children. They both suggest that the disordered groups exhibited a VOT phoneme boundary which, although correctly placed along the continuum, was not as sharp as that displayed by normally articulating children. However, it would be useful to have more conclusive evidence of this phenomenon.

Other techniques for use with DAD

1. In her *Adapted Cuing Technique*, Klick (1985) relies on the creation of manually presented visual cues which accompany orally presented speech. This method has been designed to enhance oral stimuli and increase the frequency of correct responses. The clinician uses manual gestures to represent the movements and positions required to produce consonants and vowels. The spatial dimension is given due importance. While the client is attempting speech the clinician is using her/his fingers to indicate the nasal/oral quality and the oral position (front, middle or back) of the place of articulation. Vowels are also cued according to their position and degree of openness. The cuing takes place near to and along the side of the face.

2. Chumpelik (1984) used the work of Edna Hill Younge (who in 1938 devised a method called the moto-kinaesthetic approach which depended on a series of tactile cues to promote articulatory placement) on which to base her *Prompt System* which has developed completely new prompts for each English phoneme. It is claimed to embody in its use co-articulation processes related to polysyllabic words and phrases. It also lends itself to facilitating speech production in children with sequencing errors in connected speech. Chumpelik claims that the system initiates phoneme production in children with severe unintelligibility. It uses 'patterns of neuromuscular responses' and imposes 'target articulatory movement' on the child, thereby reducing inadequate feedback and allowing for correct/processes/rules/motor responses to be formed or continued.

Experience indicates that both the Klick and the Chumpelik approach could be helpful in cases of IAP of any degree of severity. However, in severe DAD neither is likely to improve a severely dysfunctioning motor planning process.

3. Jaffe (1984) recommends *Melodic Intonation Therapy* which has been successfully used by adults with acquired dyspraxia. This technique focuses on the formulation of propositional expressive language through use of intoned sequences. Jaffe suggests that there are three reasons why this technique could succeed with developmental articulatory dyspraxia:
   a. speech production may be improved by alterations in prosody rhythm stress and intonation;
   b. emphasis on movement may improve phonemic and linguistic sequencing through intersystemic organization;
   c. the reduced rate of verbal input and verbal output may facilitate correct articulatory placement and inclusion.

From reports of previous work with children with DAD using this method it is agreed that although very young children may derive little benefit, ideal candidates are aged 7;0 to 8;0 with a moderate DAD and poor repetition skills. Use of at least three to four words and an average attention span are further requirements. The children are taught to self-cue through intonation and signing to facilitate linguistic sequencing.

4. The *Nuffield Dyspraxia Programme* is widely used in the UK. Unfortunately, this admirable programme which has proved helpful in the treatment of DAD has been misused as treatment for phonological disorders for which it was never intended. It is primarily a method for treating articulation disorders. As an articulation drill it succeeds, but a criticism is that it relies too much on the auditory channel and does not always present examples appropriate to features such as 'voicing', e.g. /k/ as the sound for 'gun'. The programme has been produced over time by the team treating children at the Nuffield Speech and Hearing Centre, London.

Once again it is important to repeat that DAD is a disorder of articulation which will affect the development of phonology but which needs to be specifically treated as a breakdown in neurophysiological development and not as a breakdown in linguistic development. Similarly, phonology is a component of language, a cognitive concept, not to be dealt with by physical drilling and repetitive exercise. DAD is a disorder of production and therefore encoding. Phonological disorders are breakdowns in decoding. Speech therapy approaches to each are therefore diametrically opposed.

If there is pathological DAD present the child will be unable to produce consistent, correct responses and the exercise may then be regarded as having been helpful in determining that other treatment approaches are required. A complicating factor can be that a child is so immature that he/she fails to succeed in these exercises and may be misdiagnosed DAD. Usually there are other contributing factors in such cases which alert the clinician to a much wider malfunctioning than only in the area of speech, e.g. poor digital motor control, delayed or deviant language use. As already mentioned, many children with DAD, if not all, have degrees of immaturity co-existing with their basic motor planning problem, thus treatment usually proves useful to some extent. An alternative system of communication may prove psychologically useful during the treatment period to increase the child's overall interactive ability.

5. Other approaches for the amelioration of DAD have been mentioned elsewhere. For example, Roach and Hardcastle (1974) record an instance when they fitted a girl of 14;0, with normal hearing and a high level of auditory discrimination, with a dental plate with 14 contacts. The only abnormal movements discernible were 'erratic and inept' movements of her tongue during fluent speech. On the assumption that she had a distorted sensory feedback loop system, the plate was devised and after several days the girl was able to control and improve her intelligibility significantly. Improvement was maintained over time. The lack of a reliable feedback system may well have resulted from DAD.

Chappell (1973, 1984) recommends attaining a 'key word vocabulary' for baseline use by each child with DAD.

EFFECT OF DAD ON CHILD PHONOLOGIES

Careful assessment of the child's phonology and syntax, possibly with the use of PACS (Grunwell, 1985) and LARSP (Crystal *et al.*, 1976), should be made at regular intervals. Severe DAD and IAP will both affect the language development of children. DAD causes the development of disordered phonology, while IAP delays phonological development to different degrees. In turn, there is often a co-occurring disorder or delay in the development of syntax. Morphology also will be affected and those children's use of language will suffer. Sometimes a child with severe DAD retains the ability to use writing and reading skills although these are generally operating at a level non-commensurate with the age of the child. Mathematics and other allied subjects may also be difficult for the child so that he/she is apparently labouring under several learning disabilities.

In Britain, many children with the constellation of symptoms which constitute DAD are referred to one of the few residential schools set up throughout the country to cater for their specific needs. However, there remain many children of school-age and over who would have benefited from much earlier diagnosis. Not only have they lost considerable ground in learning, but their parents have also contended with years of guilt, indecision and wasted time. Parents may not know *what* is wrong with their child but they do know that *something* is wrong. Too often experts do not recognize the signs, particularly of rare conditions such as DAD/IAP, nor unfortunately are they aware that referral to speech therapy may be helpful in these cases. Speech therapists have to use their knowledge, and the information which is available at this time, to facilitate early intervention. They also need to advertise their abilities much more widely, not in the commercial sense but in the form of research and relevant publications.

Experience indicates that by, at most, three years of age, and in many cases younger, there are signs which indicate a praxic breakdown for which intervention can be planned. It is *not* important at these very early stages to be absolutely sure of the final diagnosis. It *is* important that the child's unaffected abilities should be discovered and exploited to compensate for the areas of weakness which will eventually be clearly diagnosed. Voluntary Organisations Communication and Language (VOCAL) has produced a leaflet by Milloy (1988) to help parents to understand the nature of DAD and recommend initial parental handling of the situation. Parents have formed The Dyspraxia Trust to 'encourage a wider understanding of the condition' and to 'promote better diagnostic and treatment facilities' among other aims (Appendix F).

Recognition of the moderately to mildly affected child is made by acknowledging the *clumsy* child. Mild to moderate degrees of

DAD and/or IAP may be discovered when these children are assessed. In the milder cases considerable learning may take place and the amount of disadvantage to the child, his/her education and life-style, as well as to the family, may be minimal. Nevertheless, in some cases, non-recognition of the source of the child's problem may lead to misunderstandings which may grow out of all proportion to the difficulty because the child appears neither to be trying, nor to be doing his/her best work. The constraints placed on such children frequently lead to behaviour problems which alienate families and result in great misery for all involved. Some children may never be referred for speech therapy and therefore one expert who should be able to give considerable help and support may not become available.

DAD and/or IAP may co-occur with other conditions. As has been suggested, DAD and dysarthria existing in one individual may influence decisions of priorities in management. The child considered to be autistic usually has marked language difficulties. In addition, DAD may also be present. Where this is the case, the behaviour problems which arise from perceptual disintegration will be compounded by the unintelligibility created by the articulation disorder. Experience of a few such individuals has shown that this type of co-existing disability can be the factor which makes for a less acceptable appearance. Unawareness of the groping muscles and lack of appreciation of constant failure can result in the child appearing to be severely physically and mentally handicapped.

Children with severe learning disabilities occasionally have DAD. Such children can be almost totally cut off from normal social relationships. Their cognitive levels prevent them from interpreting what is going on around them and their motor dysfunction disables them from expressing their needs and desires and from attaining individual status. It is very difficult in those cases to determine where to start with intervention. This is possibly an area of neglect in speech therapy. Resources are so stretched that it is frequently the most severely disabled clients who suffer, since they require so much time both for careful and comprehensive investigation and assessment and for long-term in-depth management. It is felt that the ideal intervention strategies for this category of client is that of a well-knit team with the expertise to provide input at every possible level: social, educational, physical, occupational, linguistic and psychological, with the parents playing the focal part. It is in such circumstances that the concept of one conductor trained to meet every contingency (Peto, 1955) may provide a better approach than a group of experts who may miss some aspects of treatment and overlap in others. At present early intervention and parental support are provided in many parts of the UK by teams, including teachers and speech therapists, who carry out programmes such as The Portage Guide to Early Education (Bluma et al., 1976).

In North America, workers in this field have looked at other aspects of dyspraxia. For example, David et al. (1981), representing The Child Neurology Task Force on the Nosology of Higher Cortical Dysfunction in Children, introduced the term 'speech programming deficit syndrome'. This described children with severe oral-verbal deficits but adequate auditory comprehension. In 1982, Rapin used the term 'phonologic programming deficit syndrome' (PPDS). This assumes the initial phonetic fragmentation and starts at the first stage of the linguistic problem which results from the motor programming dysfunction. A study made by Steig Pearce et al. (1987) involved eight children with PPDS and eight normal children. It set out to evaluate learning and recall of Blissymbols and of Signed English manual signs. The results support the contention that children with PPDS not only have deficits in motor speech, but also deficits in symbolic processing. These findings indicate the effect at higher levels of language learning that articulatory motor dysfunctions may produce, or co-exist with.

No fully satisfactory solution has yet been achieved for overall management of such multiply handicapped children. It is essential, however, for society to be aware that management of such cases will be long term, perhaps with several breaks for adjustment and relaxation. Life-long support will be required in moderate and severe cases.

5

Developmental dysfluency

Fluency is the *flow* of speech. Human beings become fluent effort-lessly and automatically in the first few years of life. To signal intention, desire, dissent or whatever, human beings use the lan-guage(s) of their parents constituted by the accepted structured sequences of phonetic/phonological chunks which adhere roughly to universal rules, and which are conveyed across the ether to their listeners, by means of acoustic waves received by the latters' hearing and cognitive processes. To meet the requirements of meaning and clarity, the flow of speech should follow a prescribed form which demands no distortions or interruptions other than acceptable pauses and variations of speed. Individuals unable to meet these requirements may, as has already been reported, have various disorders and deficits which disable them and create unac-ceptable speech production. Other individuals have difficulty in maintaining the necessary flow of speech production which con-tributes to easy communicative interchange. Those people are referred to as either stammerers, stutterers or the dysfluent. For this discussion the term stutterers will be used.

Ever since it was realized that human beings used a linguistic communicative system there have been reports of stuttering. It has often been stated that there are as many theories and therapies about stuttering as there are stutterers. This situation has not changed. Basically there is controversy about whether stuttering is a problem of speech or of personality; of a neurological nature or a psychological; of childhood or of whole-life duration. What-ever the issues and implications, the fact remains that some chil-dren develop this exasperating, and sometimes crippling, defect and are plagued by it in many different ways. For many years researchers have been aware that parents play a crucial role in the development and apparent seriousness of many children's stutters.

NON-FLUENCY

A stage of non-fluency takes place in the normal speech development of many children. The relaxed parent is often heard to remark that the child is either 'thinking faster than he can speak' or 'tripping over his tongue in his enthusiasm to tell some tall tale or other'. This reaction, often accompanied by a laugh, enables a child to catch up with whatever it is that has knocked her/his thinking and speech out of synchronization, and allows her/him to pass through another developmental stage, without difficulty. For the child with over-anxious parents, however, who construe the hesitancy or repetition as the beginning of stuttering, a quite different scene is set. Nothing builds up quicker than tension and anxiety and few parents are aware of the ease with which they transfer their own anxiety to their child.

It is hard enough being unable to make oneself clear when trying to speak, without the additional feelings of guilt and failure which develop when you feel you have let your parents down. Being instructed to 'slow down and try again' only draws attention to the difficulty and makes children so self-conscious that they may react in one of several unfortunate ways. Some children withdraw and avoid talking. Others rush in, using less time and care than previously, and finish up with a greater problem than ever. If so pre-disposed, some children actually go on to develop a true stutter. Again, consideration should be given to the fact that there *is* a stage of normal non-fluency and parents-to-be should be made aware of it. It is not only parents who may precipitate a child into such a position but other adults around the child, no matter how well-meaning, may make her/him acutely aware of a condition which could be, if ignored, short-lived and unimportant. Non-fluency usually takes the form of repetition of the beginning of words. Occasionally there may be a degree of hesitancy present but this is rare.

DYSFLUENCY

Stuttering, in its full form, may become much more dramatic and include prolonging segments and syllables of production; blocking, or making hard contact, which involves obstruction to the airflow due to abnormally high tension in the articulatory and/or laryngeal muscles; avoidance strategies; accompanying tics, grimaces and other idiosyncratic features which may interfere with fluency. In this context stuttering can be seen as a disorder in the production as well as in the flow of speech. It is with this aspect of the problem that the present discussion is concerned.

Many workers have concerned themselves with the study of dysfluency, not least professional people who are also stutterers. Johnson (1959) and Van Riper (1971) are probably the best known of these. Varieties of treatment are as rife as exponents of theories on stuttering. There are those convinced that the habit of stuttering arises from an identifiable psychological problem such as conflict as propounded by Sheehan (1975), others who account for the difficulty as basically a neurological breakdown (Fransella, 1972) and yet others who feel that the problem is a 'complex interrelationship between many factors' (Andrews and Harris, 1964). Sheehan claimed that difficulties experienced in the past influence the stuttering produced in the future. Later versions of his theory emphasize 'role-conflict', indicating that stuttering arises only in particular situations or 'roles' (Sheehan and Martyn, 1970). Wischner (1969), like Johnson (1959), believes that it is parents' attitudes in relation to non-fluency which set up the reaction of anxiety in the child. In turn, the anxiety – the expectancy – leads to delaying and avoidance behaviours which are adopted to act as a barrier between the child and the displeasure of her/his listeners. Bloodstein (1960a, 1960b, 1961) describes four recognizable phases through which a child passes (recorded as similar to those of others) in the development of dysfluency.

1. The episodic phase, in which fluency is common, but dysfunction occurs mostly in the form of repetition of initial sounds in words, particularly function words, e.g. prepositions, pronouns and conjunctions.
2. The chronic phase, in which there is considerable stuttering, by this stage, primarily in content words. The child continues to be little perturbed by the stutter, except in severe cases or in instances of considerable difficulty.

71

3. The full stuttering phase without the inclusion of avoidance, although there may be exasperation and annoyance. The full emotional involvement has not yet developed.
4. The emotive phase, in which embarrassment, fear, self-consciousness and other undermining feelings are evoked, both by the struggle for fluency by the child and the difficulty in understanding, experienced by his/her listener.

Although these facile phases do not fully describe or cover the gamut of distress and disruption suffered in dysfluency they do outline the recognizable stages through which the child passes. In 1970, Bloodstein himself, with a greater awareness of linguistic development, changed the details of his phases, but on the whole, he has maintained the original outline.

Van Riper (1971), disagreeing with both Bloodstein's phases and his own previous concepts of stages of stuttering, proposes 'certain common patterns of progressive change'. He describes a situation which places less emphasis on psychological aspects of behaviour and more on the possibility that a neurophysiological event is being experienced. After studying 300 stutterers longitudinally, he observes that the majority of them recover from their early difficulties and achieve fluency leaving a small number with a continuing problem. This fact can be compared with the situation recently revealed in the development of praxis (Milloy, 1985). The question arises as to the maturational implications in the cases of children with early problems which eventually become resolved. Further research is urgently required to elucidate the understanding of the motor, emotional and related problems undergone by a not inconsiderable number of children in their efforts to develop normal speech production.

Evidence exists that neural events are altered just prior to articulation (McClean, 1977; Smith and Luschei, 1983), and that measuring these events in children who stutter produces results showing increases in reflex movements depending on the severity of the stutter. Peters (1986) discerns a link between stuttering and dis-coordination of motor activity within different subsystems of the speech mechanism. Indications of a right hemisphere involvement for speech is claimed by Moore and Haynes (1980). In a different context, Van Riper (1971) makes an interesting observation in which he states that

when a person stutters on a word there is a temporal disruption of the simultaneous and successive programming of muscular movements required to produce one of the word's integrated sounds, or to emit one of its syllables appropriately
or to accomplish the precise linking of sounds and syllables
that constitutes its motor pattern. If we ignore for the
moment the entire complex overlay of reactions to this experience, we find the essence of the disorder in this fracturing
and disruption of the motor sequencing of the word. The
integrity of a spoken word demands great precision in the
timing of its components. When for any reason, that timing
is awry and askew, a temporally distorted word is produced,
and when this happens the speaker has evinced a core stuttering behaviour.

(p. 404)

This pronouncement poses several problems. In the first place, it
acknowledges once more the critical role of timing in the actual
production of speech. Timing is implicit in programming for movement of the groups of muscles used to operate the organs of
articulation. Only by employing a finely graded timing mechanism
can the precise, clean muscle movements be made which produce
intelligibility. Van Riper actually uses the word 'programming'
with reference to his description of the disruption of integrated
sounds. But programming of movements is surely reminiscent of
the basis of praxis, and the disruption of such programming is
surely the description of dyspraxia. Is it true then that stuttering
and dyspraxia are synonymous or is one a causal factor of the
other?

STUTTERING v. DYSPRAXIA

In 1980, Rosenbek discussed the relationship of stuttering and
apraxia of speech (his term). He has concentrated most of his
work in the adult area, but occasionally he refers to the developmental when discussing early pathology. Rosenbek reviews the
work of several experts and concludes that there is sufficient
evidence to support the theory that there may be a close affinity
between stuttering and some forms of dyspraxia (Luria, 1966;
Wingate, 1967; Trost, 1971; Caplan, 1972). Caplan concludes,
after studying the dysfluencies in the speech of several dysphasics,

that stuttering may be a form of dyspraxia. He drew parallels between stuttering and both ideational and ideomotor dyspraxia. It is possible to describe developmental articulatory dyspraxia (DAD) as a form of ideomotor dyspraxia.

Most of these studies apply to adult patients, but it is clear that similar conditions may be found in the course of developmental stages to those acquired due to disease or trauma in later life. At a later stage in his review Rosenbek discusses dyspraxia as a cause of stuttering. Many writers have tried to localize the site of lesion in dyspraxia. Experience indicates the inadvisability of this as there is indubitable evidence of inconsistency in DAD which includes the occasional production of correctly produced segments, syllables, words, phrases and sentences. This fact indicates that DAD should be regarded as a result of dysfunction of part of the brain and not of damage which can be specifically localized. This, in turn, makes Van Riper's claim for his timing hypothesis very tempting as an explanation of at least one cause of stuttering. Rosenbek postulates another hypothesis, that 'stuttering may be an adaptive response to apraxic errors'. He sees the need for more than apraxia *per se* to explain stuttering and suggests that the desire to be correct may be the missing component. In adult cases of dysphasia this may be cogent but a great deal more research than is available at present is required to make the same claims for the relationship between dyspraxia and stuttering, at developmental stages. The references to loci of errors is not convincing with regard to the claim that word-initial sounds or syllables are more frequently affected than word-final sounds or syllables for two reasons. Firstly, in moderate and severe cases of both DAD and stuttering all loci present with difficulty. Also, as the language used becomes more complex, the struggle to produce it intelligibly increases.

Kent (1985) suggests that stutterers and non-stutterers differ in that the former have less or no capacity to generate temporal programmes, or action time structures. Whereas dyspraxia may arise from the lack of a motor programme leading to the absence of feedback, Kent thinks that the temporal programme he envisages may be lacking in stutterers thus disrupting their perceptual processing of sequences, their ability to regulate motor sequences and their ability to establish effective feedback.

It does seem likely that there may be some interrelationship between the two as shared actions have been recorded and similar symptoms can be recognized.

Children who stutter are frequently thought to be delayed in language and speech development evincing early articulation difficulties (Andrews *et al.*, 1983).

Management

To treat stuttering, speech therapists have devised more techniques and approaches than for any other defect of speech production. The recorded failure rate is also the highest. This is possibly due to the fact that there have always been so many different opinions about the nature of the problem. Children with any deficit in speech production which does not respond to straightforward muscular drills are difficult clients to deal with, as their life experience is limited and it is not easy either to work in areas which have become charged with both emotional pressure and frequent failure or to discuss unformed attributes such as 'feelings' and 'attitudes'. The personal constructs approach (Fransella, 1970), which may be relevant for use with older children and adults, does not lend itself to use with younger children.

Traditional relaxation approaches are also very difficult to convey to the very young. In fact, for these children, experience indicates that it is the behaviour of the adults surrounding them that is of greatest importance and help. This behaviour should be geared to provide an easy, non-restrictive but constant routine with kindly, firm discipline and reliable support.

In the UK current trends favour as early identification and intervention as possible. A tradition has arisen in which many authorities run groups for intensive therapy with children who stutter. The techniques employed are eclectic, dependent on the previous successes of the speech therapists running the group. In addition, practice is included in groups and individually of everyday situations which have become problematic in the normal course of living. Such situations may include using the 'phone, asking for a bus ticket, shopping, etc.

A similar programme of intensive treatment for both parents and children, including younger, pre-school children is described overleaf.

Clinical techniques

Specific approaches have been devised to assess and treat pre-school children who have disordered fluency. Culp (1984) designed The Pre-school Fluency Development Programme to meet the needs of children whom she felt were being neglected with respect to their development of fluency. Samples of the children's everyday use of speech are obtained by means of assessment procedures. Comparison is made qualitatively and quantitatively with the speech of normally fluent children of the same age group. The programme focuses on the integration of hierarchies of fluency, in which attempts are made to establish fluency through exercises with words, phrases and sentences. At each level seven stages are practised as follows:

Establishing fluency

1. choral speaking
2. clinician provides immediate model
3. clinician provides immediate model in a disruptive situation
4. clinician provides a delayed model
5. clinician provides a delayed model in a disruptive situation
6. child produces spontaneously
7. child produces spontaneously in a disruptive situation.

Generalizing fluency in connected speech

1. story completion (gradually increasing mean length of response)
   a. play setting
   b. disruptive setting
   c. home setting (optional)
2. monologue (1–3 above)
3. dialogue (1–3 above).

Running concurrently with the programme, Culp has planned an individualized parent training scheme which involves 7 hours of direct contact, which can be arranged in various blocks of time but which takes place during the first 2 months of the child's programme. The first of the three components of this training consists of seven basic units:

1. explanatory introduction
2. analysis of frequently reported dysfluent episodes
3. recording fluency at home
4. child development
5. discipline
6. helping the child express feelings
7. review.

Secondly, monthly observations of the children in therapy are arranged. Parents report that this is most helpful in applying fluency techniques at home and recognizing their child's progress. Finally, the parent training includes the parents' maintenance group which meets twice monthly and helps to maintain interest, to review fluency facilitation skills and to solve new problems as they arise.

Culp claims several reasons for the therapeutic effectiveness of her programme. The first of these is the direct child therapy supported by parent training and focuses on hierarchies of fluency, child and linguistic environment. A further effective contribution is the consistent introduction of fluency disruptors in therapy to ensure equivalence to real-life settings. Also, the influence of positive feedback in enjoyable communication experiences appear to enhance each child's fluency and general development. Advantages of the therapy are:

1. the inclusion of a reliable assessment procedure for individuals' fluency evaluation and for comparison with normative data;
2. the flexibility of the programme in terms of materials required and the option of individual or group therapy and parent and/or teacher training;
3. the documentation which provides strong support for wider clinical use.

The Culp approach is similar in some respects to the Monterey Fluency Programme which was devised by Bruce Ryan and Barbara van Kirk, and works through reading, monologue and conversation. When fluency has been achieved at each level the client progresses to the transfer and maintenance programmes. These then use the 'speak more freely' approach. Contrary approaches consider how clients may 'stutter more fluently' (Van Riper, 1973). This is regarded as a very much more personalized approach where individual treatment is the order of the day.

The Assessment and Therapy Programme for Dysfluent Children (Rustin, 1987) includes parents and their children who stutter and covers a two-week period in which a daily weekday programme is carried out after comprehensive assessment and evaluation has taken place of the children's speech and contributing factors supplied by the parents/carers.

Byrne (1983) produced a book full of useful information for people concerned with people who stutter, and for the stutterers themselves. She covers a wide area when citing the possible therapies for stuttering, favouring none in particular but suggesting, as many therapists do, that there is a need for many approaches to meet the idiosyncratic requirements of many different types of people who stutter. Both child and adult approaches are included. She mentions such opposing ideas as: slow/prolonged speech; syllable-timed speech; the airflow technique; relaxation, hypnosis, yoga, meditation; drug therapies such as sedatives, tranquillizers; personal constructs and psychotherapy.

Claims of considerable successes in treating child stuttering are made by Riley and Riley (1984). They tend to agree with the notion of familial diathesis in cases of child stutterers. This was mentioned by Morley (1972). Trait(s) for some language/speech weakness can apparently be inherited. The form(s) of language/-speech difficulty may then vary, within the possible gamut of such disorders, from child to child. However, it is often possible to trace at least one other stutterer in an extended family. Since the ratio of stuttering consistently presents at 3:1 to 4:1 male to female, it is often easier to monitor the more frequent lines of male descent for such succeeding stutterers.

Riley and Riley assess the speech of young children using procedures devised by themselves for the purpose. Parents and their attitudes to their child's stutter play an important role in the management programme. The four major areas of their model are modification of:

1. the environment
2. the child's attitude
3. any neurological components
4. remaining abnormal dysfluencies.

The sequence is varied from individual to individual according to her/his needs. Reduction of parent guilt and anxiety are paramount in the overall approach and careful, comprehensive parent counselling is set in motion. Parent attitudes are discussed and attempts made to enable parents to modify them and to adopt a reasonable level of expectation of the child's behaviour, including her/his fluency, which need not be perfect. With respect to the speech production aspects, these experts pay particular attention to what they term oral motor discoordination. They 'view oral motor timing as a feed-forward, motor planning process aimed at an acoustic target' (p. 153). This categorizes them as yet other workers who are drawing parallels between stuttering and praxis, although they do not mention this fact *per se*. They go on to say:

> We theorize that improved motor planning tends to normalize voice onset and termination times and to improve transitional formants. If this is so the child's fluent speech should improve and the modification of remaining stuttering events should be simpler.
>
> (p. 153)

Intervention must be undertaken at the earliest possible age according to Riley and Riley. In fact they claim that if every child who exhibits chronic abnormal dysfluencies could begin treatment within a few months of stuttering onset, almost all stuttering could be eliminated before the primary school years. They are particularly incensed by the idea which persists in some areas that children with dysfluency will 'grow out of it'.

Another American speech pathologist who strongly advocates early intervention for young stuttering children is Shine (1984). He claims to start his treatment with children as young as three years of age and his particular mentors were Van Riper (1973), Ryan (1974) and Wingate (1976). His fluency training programme includes physiological, prosodic and linguistic aspects. He employs token economy to maintain motivation and also takes specific passing/failing criteria into account. Two of his aims are to achieve a 'fluent speaking mode' and an 'easy speaking voice'. The former involves the child in practice using either whispered speech, prolonged speech or both while the latter concentrates on the establishment of normal pause, easy onset, continuous airflow, a normal prosodic pattern and the unstressed form of strong/weak forms. Child and parent attitudes and awareness are also worked on and transfer and maintenance of improved fluency sought. Shine claims that a 5-year follow-up of this direct fluency training approach reveals that young children are able to establish and maintain normally fluent speaking patterns with rare instances of recurrent stuttering. These and other researchers (Costello, 1983; Rustin *et al.*, 1987) go a long way to refute previous claims that intervention in the very early years was deleterious for children with dysfluency. It should be repeated, however, that care should be taken to determine that one is not dealing with normal non-fluency.

CLUTTERING

Although there is strictly no absolute comparison between stuttering and cluttering, there is a sufficient resemblance between the two to consider the effect of cluttering on speech production at this juncture. Historically, Weiss (1964) was the greatest authority on cluttering. His definition of the condition is here presented in full.

> Cluttering is a speech disorder characterised by the clutterer's unawareness of his disorder, by a short attention span, by disturbances in perception, articulation and formulation of speech and often by speed of delivery. It is a disorder of the thought process preparatory to speech and based on a hereditary disposition. Cluttering is the verbal manifestation of Central Language Imbalance, which affects all channels of communication (e.g. Reading, writing, rhythm and musicality) and behavior in general.
>
> (p. 1)

From the productive level, cluttering is usually first observed by the rapid delivery (tachylalia), although sometimes slowed delivery (bradylalia) is presented. The child who clutters has a recognizable life-style which includes imprecise attempts at all motor and linguistic skills. Wolk (1986) presents a case study of a male adult who at the age of 12;0 was noticed by his schoolteacher to have a speech disorder. He was described as scruffy, awkward and immature. His mother and brother also had cluttering-like symptoms. The boy completed his secondary and tertiary schooling and was employed as a cost accountant. Fourteen years after the first referral, at age 26;0, his employer referred him once more for investigation. Once again he was described as untidy, clumsy and fidgety. He was totally unaware of and unconcerned about his speech. Eventually he was diagnosed as a clutterer according to Diedrich's (1984) five characteristic features. These are:

1. diagnosis of cluttering usually confirmed around C.A. 7;0;
2. impaired language function – dissociation between thinking and speaking;
3. speech disorder (either/or/all)
   a. unintelligibility
   b. dysfluency
   c. lack of self-awareness
   d. monotonous melody-rhythm;
4. lack of self-awareness;
5. hereditary or familial;

Diedrich describes the speech disorder as resulting from a lack of co-ordination between breathing and phonation with a tendency for hypernasal resonance. He points out that one useful diagnostic characteristic of cluttering that distinguishes it from other speech disorders is the use of slow and exaggerated movements of articulation. Comparable articulatory movement is not observed in developmental dysarthria, developmental articulatory dyspraxia (DAD) or phonological disorders. Experience has not revealed this tendency, but extensive study with numerous cluttering cases has not been possible so such a sign may well be apparent in some subjects. Misarticulation of sounds, particularly sibilants and liquids is also mentioned by Diedrich. He concludes that the speech disorders issue from a problem of self-monitoring speech output. The overall difficulties are regarded by Diedrich as being comparable to a language learning disorder with disruption of the central language process as the basis of the problem.

Wolk used this subject to explore the use of Luria's Neuropsych ological Investigation (LNI) and a dichotic consonant-vowel (CV) listening task. The results revealed on the LNI suggested symptomatology consistent with a lesion in the left fronto-temporal division. This was confirmed on the electroencephalogram. Findings from the CV listening task indicated possible disturbances in both auditory processing and in place perception. There continues to be controversy regarding the prognosis for clutterers.

Dalton and Hardcastle (1977) appear to suggest that improvement is possible but difficult, and depends on the application of each particular clutterer. Diagnosis should be completed and management should be well under way before adolescence according to Diedrich (1984). As with other types of rare condition, e.g. DAD, cluttering is complex in nature, presenting with many variables and creating numerous problems of diagnosis and management. However, these two conditions are not dissimilar except for the one major difference that the DAD sufferer is well aware of failure and the ineffectiveness of her/his attempts to communicate, while the clutterer appears to feel that his/her communicative system is totally adequate.

Management

Treatment for cluttered speech takes similar lines to that for stuttering. Slowed speech, rhythmic and shadowing exercises, exaggerated articulation, prosodic exercises particularly for stressing and phrasing are included. In addition, space, time and location should be explored in connection with whole-body awareness and positioning, limb and head positioning and, of course, oral mechanism awareness. The adapted Cuing Technique formulated by Klick (1985) could also be applied, as could all the proprioceptive and visual cues used in the treatment of DAD and IAP. At least half of the management will be concentrated on language aspects, particularly those concerned with sequencing, deixis and such necessary areas.

Reading, writing, spelling and design may also require specific work to improve the prognosis. The level at which these can be applied will depend on the ability and motivation of the individual. Weiss (1964) states that in cluttering the chances of self-improvement are tenuous since the typical clutterer is unaware of his/her problem. This can be rectified to some extent when the client hears his/her speech on tape. Improvement has been noted when exercises for speed and clarity are carried out on audiotape enabling the client to repair and repeat in the process of practice. It is still uncertain whether generalization can be achieved using this method.

Diedrich claims that a marked improvement has been noted when clutterers attend to their own speech by using a slow exaggerated pattern. He points out that this monitoring does not appear to improve the child's language formulation, however.

6

Developmental voice disorders

Early vocal behaviour in neonates signals initial reciprocal communicative exchanges. Parents are programmed to respond to the most primitive of infantile attempts and very quickly establish the basis for turn-taking by construing simplistic forms of sound-making as equivalents to adult speech forms. This is the beginning of language development which is possibly the most important human skill learnt by infants during their years of dependence. Language is species specific to *homo sapiens* and no matter how much one tries it appears impossible to teach more than the most fundamental elements of language to other species, however high up the evolutionary scale they may be. Language, of course, has many aspects. Facial expression, for example, is an observable aspect which is present at a quite early stage of human development, with eye contact and vocalization. The three together seem to be the start of bonding a young infant into his/her specific group.

Other skills occur concurrently which are closely associated with that of developing vocalization. For example, at a relatively early stage a baby is able to locate the source of sound set up by his/her mother's voice, and will respond to it by turning his/her head towards it. These signs of early recognition and response emphasize the centrality of sight and sound in human communication. They draw attention to the fact that the selection of speech sounds from the cacophony of environmental 'noise' also takes place early. Infants appear to be programmed to listen to, learn from and eventually use, in a primitive fashion, the dominant mode of communication with which they are surrounded, their 'mother tongue'.

Considerable work has been done on the isolation of sounds made by infants using displays produced by sound level recorders, laryngographs and electromyographs (Martin, 1981; Stemple, 1984). Normal voice development is outlined by Aronson (1985). He describes the changing position and structure of the larynx at birth, through infancy, childhood and puberty until adulthood. One area in which a great deal of research has been carried out is that of determining the variation of cries used in infancy. For example, Wasz-Hockert *et al.* (1968) obtained evidence from listeners of four distinctive types of cries from birth to seven months:

1. birth signal: *c.* 1 sec. in duration; flat or falling melody; usually voiceless; always strained or strident; contains glottal plosives;
2. pain signal: long duration; usually falling melody; high-pitched; strident;
3. hunger signal: pitch rising-falling; frequent glottal plosives;
4. pleasure signal: hypernasal; greater pitch variability than the other types of cries; rare glottal plosives; never voiceless; never strident.

Cries illustrate at a very early age that the true and false vocal folds respond differentially, depending upon the individual's psychophysiological state. The strained, harsh, tense cry of pain is forced owing to massive, tight closure of the laryngeal tract. This means that it is an undifferentiated adduction of both true and false vocal folds. The pleasure cry is lax, more sonorous, and devoid of strain and effort and produced only by the true vocal folds. Wasz-Hockert *et al.* asked 349 women to identify and categorize 24 infant birth, pain, hunger and pleasure cries. Results indicated that pleasure cries were identified most accurately followed by hunger, pain and birth cries. It was interesting to note that the accuracy of judgements was dependent on the rater's background. In rank order the listeners were:

1. midwives
2. children's nurses
3. mothers
4. registered nurses
5. women experienced in child care
6. women with no experience in child care.

Hollien and Muller (1973) queried the results of Wasz-Hockert's study and set up an opposing study to ascertain whether

1 Birth and pleasure vocalizations should not have been juxtaposed.
2. Preselection of 'typical' samples of cries for listener judgements may have biased the listeners.
3. Cry duration and infant age ought to have been controlled experimentally and statistically.

They designed a study in which they recorded cries stimulated by pain, noise and hunger from eight infants: four females and four males aged between 3 and 5 months. Two groups of listeners were used: the mothers of the eight children, and mothers of similarly aged infants. Results showed that the acoustic characteristics of normal infants' cries carry little perceptual information to the mother about the reasons for the cries. However, the experimenters felt little confidence in the outcome and do not set too much store by it. It seems important that so little certainty is still felt about this situation, thus the aforementioned information has been detailed, and the need for further research into the area emphasized.

With regard to voice fundamental frequency, it seems that 300 to 400 Hz above the adult average is recorded in infancy. Facial expression appears to be inseparable from infant cries. Intonation is also noted at an early stage in development. Dropping of the fundamental frequency of the voice towards the end of a sustained utterance is recorded at the earliest stages. Thus there appears to be an innate physiological basis for intonation. It has long been accepted that infants respond to intonation before they are able to comprehend language (Lewis, 1936).

When explaining how normal phonation occurs it is necessary to have two surfaces, one resistant to the other so that when they strike vibration results. To produce voice, the reservoir of air pressure striking the resistant vocal folds creates vibrations which are resonated in the chest, pharynx, nose, mouth and the sinuses. Since size, shape and anatomical dimensions vary from person to person, each individual voice is intrinsically different. It is how the breath and the resonators are used that is important. They should be used to the best advantage by each individual.

The fundamental frequency of the human voice descends with age, particularly between birth and adolescence, paralleling the descent of the larynx in the neck. Complete documentation of the levels of descent are not available but Fairbanks *et al.* (1949) recorded the mean fundamental frequency of seven-year-olds as 286.5 Hz while McGlone and McGlone (1972) found that in eight-year-olds to be 275.8 Hz. A more recent investigation (Sorenson, 1989) tested fundamental frequencies of 30 children aged between 6;0 and 10;0. Results showed that the average fundamental frequencies of females was 262 Hz. Males scored 281 Hz. This is a non-significant difference.

CONGENITAL VOICE DISORDERS

Vocal fold lesions

Neonates who are ill or have a specific voice disorder will sound different from normal when they cry. For example, the Cri du Chat syndrome is so-called because of the distinctive, high-pitched, cat-like cry of the child. Studies disclose that this disorder is due to a chromosomal defect (Ward *et al.*, 1968). Laryngeal disease or disorder frequently result in *stridor*. This means involuntary sound made during inhalation or exhalation. Neoplasms, inflammation, or other forms of abnormality may result in stridor which is often the first indication that all is not well. Different types of laryngeal defects include:

1. Laryngeal web   Around the tenth week of embryonic development the web of tissue surrounding the glottis separates. If this separation fails to take place and the web is complete, surgery will be required immediately after birth to maintain life. However, webs are most often partial and found at the level of the vocal folds. The voices of children with such webs vary, depending on the site and extent of the lesion, between hoarseness and aphonia.
2. Subglottic stenosis   This is an obstructive narrowing of the airway, usually between the vocal folds and the cricoid area, and due to arrested embryonic development will result in stridor, although crying is usually normal.
3. Laryngotracheal cleft   A rare condition caused by embryonic failure of fusion of the dorsal cricoid lamina which leads to an interarytenoid cleft and an open larynx posteriorly. The feeding problems created frequently overshadow voice difficulties.

4. Inflammation   This may take several forms, e.g. laryngitis, croup after diphtheria, bronchitis, epiglottitis, and can cause aphonia or dysphonia according to severity.
5. Malnutrition   Specific cries are identifiable in infants who are malnourished. They have been compared with the cries of infants with central nervous system disease.
6. Syndromes   For example, syndromes recently recognized, such as fetal alcohol syndrome and that resulting from maternal drug abuse, appear to affect vocalizations in the newly born. Down's syndrome may also present with vocal anomalies.
7. Papillomata   These most common laryngeal growths of childhood are occasionally to be found in neonates. It is thought that they are caused by specific viral infections and, despite repeated surgical intervention, they can recur persistently. These benign lesions usually regress with age and disappear during puberty. Depending on the size and location of the masses there may be hoarseness in mild cases and aphonia in the most severe cases. Other growths which may erupt along the length of vocal folds are nodes or nodules, warts or cysts.
8. Carcinoma   Occasionally, infants are born with, or develop at an early stage, malignant neoplasms affecting the vocal folds and so detectable in the vocalizations. Somewhat older children may also present with cancers which involve voice production. These conditions are rare.
9. Trauma   Infantile larynxes are subject to internal or external trauma, which will have an effect on vocalization.

Neurological disorders

For normal cries to be emitted neonates should have reached a certain state of maturity neurologically. In the presence of different types of neurological disease, disorder or immaturity, the quality of vocalization used by infants will be affected, depending on the nature, site and severity of the lesion. Infectious, neoplastic, vascular and/or degenerative disease may be responsible for different types of vocal anomalies. As Aronson (1985) points out:

neurologic voice disorders, technically, are dysarthrias; although they occur in isolation, most often they are imbedded in a more widespread complex of respiratory, resonatory, and articulatory dysarthric signs.

(p. 77)

Infancy

Cries are usually high-pitched, shrill, weak and unsustained. Duration of cries is abnormally short. Xth (vagus) nerve lesions causing unilateral or bilateral paralysis leads to abnormal crying, which may involve one or several cranial nerves. Adductor vocal fold paralysis results in weak or absent cries. Alternatively, bilateral abductor paralysis may leave the voice and cry normal due to adequate approximation of the vocal folds. However, inhalatory stridor may be present because the vocal folds are too weak to be abducted during inhalation.

Childhood

Children may develop any or most of the disorders which affect adults. The respiratory, phonatory and/or articulatory involvement will result in hoarse, breathy, weak and/or festinating production of voice, while intonation may be affected due to imbalance of nasality. Pitch, stress, volume and all aspects of prosody may be absent or disrupted in such conditions and the overall presentation of vocalization and eventually productive language may be severely enough affected to interfere with and reduce intelligibility. Self-monitoring to facilitate the development of phonology may be unreliable and normal speech will not develop.

As in adulthood, the specific type of dysarthria depends on site, severity, etc. The type of dysarthria dictates the nature of the resultant dysphonia. Thus, cortical involvement leading to spastic dysarthria, extrapyramidal involvement leading to athetoid or rigid dysarthria, and cerebellar involvement leading to ataxic dysarthria, will have a different effect on the type, nature and severity of dysphonia which will be present. Children with some degree of cerebral palsy are frequently liable to have voice disorders. Supra- or generalized bulbar palsy results from damage to several cranial nerves. In addition to the involvement of the articulators, the vocal folds are seen to be weak on examination, affecting voice production. In particular, damage to the Xth (vagus) nerve results in flaccid dysphonia. The normal function of this nerve is to close the glottis for voiced sounds and open it for unvoiced sounds. Left or right unilateral vagal paralysis results in fixation of the corresponding vocal fold in an abducted position at or near the midline. If the former is the case, the voice is usually harsh, breathy and reduced in volume. If fixed near the midline, the voice will be harsh and reduced in loudness. In both cases, diplophonia, inhalatory stridor and short phrases may be observed. Monotony of both pitch and loudness may also be noted.

Other causes

Children with cleft palate(s) relatively frequently have vocal problems secondary to the primary condition. In this case it is the velopharyngeal insufficiency which leads to the use of characteristic hypernasal vocal qualities. A disturbance in normal vocal resonance is discernible in children who are hard-of-hearing. It is thought that this results from their tendency to speak with a tongue position retracted towards the pharyngeal wall.

Like every other physical condition which may have an effect on the production of speech, a predisposition may exist for voice disorders, that is, the vocal folds may be one of the weak areas of an individual's physical make-up. These may then be subject to infection and/or inflammation in the presence of viruses, bacteria or other invasions. Some people always develop a severe cough when they catch cold, others have stuffed noses and sinuses and yet others lose their voices as a result of laryngitis. Occasionally children with this type of predisposition may have vocal trouble due to inability to cope with stressful situations. This usually occurs in adults but some children are so pressured that dysphonia develops which is difficult to account for in any other way. This should not be confused with 'selective' or 'elective' mutism, which is a condition in which no organic voice disorder exists but in which a child decides not to speak at all, i.e. remain mute, in certain circumstances (see p. 96).

Some children with no obvious laryngeal weakness may develop voice problems through vocal abuse. This usually results from persistent shouting and general abuse of the vocal folds, and may be accompanied by other unsocial behaviours. This cannot be regarded primarily as a voice disorder but rather a part of a greater whole which requires investigation, usually of a psychological nature. However, perhaps the child does have the type of physical predisposition already mentioned. All of those symptoms may disappear when the cause(s) of the basic insecurity has (have) been discovered and dealt with satisfactorily, and suitable methods of vocal use have been learned and adopted. In some children, however, the repeated shouting creates nodules or nodes on the vocal folds which need surgical removal.

Vocal disability in children may also arise as part of a constellation of symptoms of general debility, e.g. under-nourishment, neglect and generally poor environmental conditions.

Management

The aim of therapy is to train or restore the voice to an adequate level for the client's daily needs. This is no easy task when dealing with children where it is believed that the baseline for therapy is voice rest. Some experts think that only by ceasing the use of the abusive voicing which has become a counter-productive habit will the scene be set for learning habits conducive to more desirable voice production. Others take an opposing stand, believing that clients need to adopt firm, normally loud voices produced with equally firm exhalatory force. These workers deplore the idea of voice rest.

Preliminary steps for therapy have to be taken by determining clearly what nature of vocal use has become the practice of each client. For example, in children with an accepted habit of vocal abuse resulting from persistent shouting, it is necessary to know how they shout. Stemple and Bailey (1982) demonstrated in a study that the physical characteristics of shouting varied in children with and without vocal nodules (VN). Several children, some normal and some with VN, were investigated. It was found that at normal conversational levels, children with VN yielded higher intensity, fundamental frequency and tension levels than normal children. When induced to shout VN children did not increase intensity or tension measures. However, their frequency levels were increased significantly, indicating that the presence of vocal nodules may be enhanced by the significant increase in pitch level used in shouting. Stemple and Bailey suggest that speech therapists do not always inquire about other forms of abusive voice behaviour used by many children being assessed for voice disorders. Those vocal noises may include aeroplane, car, machine-gun, sirens and other noises. In fact, some modern heroes like the Incredible Hulk roared in a way that became popular to imitate. It is beneficial to eliminate or replace with less harmful sounds those noises which may be deleterious to the vocal folds. Some families are guilty of shouting within their home environment. This is another factor which should be investigated. This, of course, relies on the cooperation and understanding of the parents.

It may be that in the development of vocal abuse the laryngeal pathology has resulted in laryngeal muscle weakness. This also has to be assessed before management can be planned. A further habit which should be screened for is that of constantly clearing the throat. This arises from perpetual attempts made by the child to rid him/herself of the feeling of obstruction which is created by mucous drainage due to, for example, colds or allergies. It also occurs in 'lump in the throat' cases where the client is convinced that there is an obstruction in his/her throat which he/she constantly tries to be rid of by clearing the throat. The persistent throat clearing attempts lead to oedema and irritation which lead to further clearing. The habit itself, if perpetuated and repeated too often, may lead in turn to a true laryngeal pathology. Stemple and Lehmann (1980) state:

> Throat clearing is one of the most abusive things you can do to your vocal folds. When you clear your throat you create an extreme amount of movement of your vocal folds, causing them to slam and rub together . . . Sometimes people do not even know that they are doing it. But often they feel that there is something in their throat like a lump or mucous. The majority of the time, however, when you clear your throat, there is simply nothing there. The only thing you have accomplished is to create more vocal fold abuse.
>
> (p. 113)

Thus prerequisites for management of vocal abuse include:

1. isolating, identifying and assessing the specific abuse(s);
2. describing the effect(s); young children can understand anatomical and physiological explanations with the use of simple diagrams and pictures;
3. outlining more useful means of vocal use to substitute for those previously adopted;
4. considering the problems of daily living and taking steps to

enable the client and his/her family to adapt better to everyday demands;

5. accepting that occasionally it is not going to be possible either to isolate and/or change the specific cause of the voice disorder;
6. tailoring the management programme to the individual.

Initial general approach

All vocal tract habits usually require modification. It is frequently necessary to employ basic exercises (BE) for this purpose. Thus, breathing, phonating and resonating exercises should be adapted to the particular needs of each child. Some form of relaxation therapy is often required to reduce the accumulated and customary tensions which regularly accompany vocal stress and disturbance (Appendix A).

Aronson (1985) discusses at length specific musculo-skeletal tension which is a frequent feature of both organic and non-organic voice disorders. Although this consideration is seen as essential in the treatment of adults with voice disorders, it can meet a need which is also present in children and may be regarded as a strong approach in preventative therapy. Aronson emphasizes that:

Vocal hyperfunction is the most important concept in the aetiology and treatment of non-organic, and many organic, voice disorders. Intrinsic and extrinsic laryngeal muscle tension expresses anxiety, depression or anger. In organic voice disorders it may occur as a result of efforts to compensate for the organic deficit. *All patients with voice disorders regardless of aetiology, should be tested for excess musculoskeletal tension, either as a primary or as a secondary cause of dysphonia.* The degree of voice improvement following therapy for musculoskeletal tension is proportional to the reduction of musculoskeletal tension.

He then gives the following principles basic to therapy for musculoskeletal tension associated with vocal hyperfunction.

1. Extrinsic and intrinsic laryngeal muscle cramping is responsible for the abnormal voice. Reducing musculoskeletal tension releases the inherent capability of the larynx to produce normal voice.

92

2. When gently rubbed or kneaded, muscles relax and become less painful.
3. Lowering laryngeal position in the neck permits more normal phonation. (p. 339)

For a technical description of the procedure to implement these principles see Aronson (1985), pp. 340–2.

Self-monitoring

After some degree of ease has been established alongside more normal habits of breathing, particular emphasis should be placed on enabling the client to hear her/his own voice production and compare it with normal voice production. In voice cases, as in most other defects in production of speech, self-monitoring of speech production is frequently faulty. Experience has shown that until specific steps have been taken to rectify this, full recovery from any speech disorder is difficult to achieve. A particular feature of recovery from voice disorder is that early in the treatment, improved voice may appear suddenly and momentarily. Although the therapist may hear and register the improvement, the client may not, unless she/he has been alerted to the possibility and also is able to distinguish between the habitual, unacceptable voice and the normal. This is one of numerous reasons why therapy sessions should be audio-taped. It is encouraging for clients to hear improvement and where this is short-lived and not recognized much useful feedback is lost.

Occasionally, a child may develop a hormonal imbalance post-operatively or due to malfunction of the endocrine system. It is interesting to note that vocal difficulties are unlikely to occur unless the child's auditory feedback system attempts to modify the pitch level back to the original level.

Pitch

In almost every case of laryngeal pathology, pitch is registered as either too high or too low. Each individual has an optimum pitch level. The decision to aim for this level in cases of voice disorder will be influenced by whether or not a physical change is deemed to be the immediate objective. For example, where surgical intervention is required to remove an intrusive mass such as papillomata, direct voice therapy to modify pitch would be counter-

93

productive. It will frequently be found that normal pitch will follow physical recovery. Direct pitch modification to try to achieve optimum pitch would be implemented where excessive shouting has caused the voice problem, which has been diagnosed before the tissue of the vocal folds has been harmed. Usually a higher pitch than that habitually adopted, is found to be appropriate. This can mostly be achieved by asking the client to 'hum' easily. Most people 'hum' at a comfortable level near to their natural pitch level. General vocal tone will be improved with the establishment of optimum pitch.

McGlone and Brown (1969) describe three vocal modes in which pitch plays a major role. The mode which allows for the highest pitches is *light voice (falsetto)*, that for middle pitches is *heavy voice (chest)*, and the lowest and least used range involves *pulsated voice (glottal fry or vocal fry)*. It is primarily the 'break' between them which permits identification of those modes. Men, women and children use heavy voice because it provides the most socially useful pitch, loudness and voicing ranges. Unfortunately, it also allows for the greatest vocal effort and constriction, the very ingredients of vocal abuse. In heavy voice the vocal muscles are thickened and used to control volume. This mode permits the widest range of fundamental frequencies and intensities, and the strongest harmonic structure. Light voice occurs physiologically when the vocal muscles are stretched, narrowed, and used to control pitch, and it permits the highest fundamental frequencies and has weak harmonic structure. Pulsated voice is produced by short relaxed vocal folds that close rapidly and maintain the closed position for a relatively long portion of each glottal cycle. Thus only very low fundamental frequencies are permitted with energy decay in each glottal pulse. This knowledge and a great deal more that is known about what can go wrong with voice production does not facilitate the therapist's attempt to put it right. There has long been a dichotomy of approaches in dealing with vocal disorders. One has focused on determining and attempting to establish natural pitch, and working on other non-segmental factors such as loudness. The second has been a concentrated holistic approach in which the rehabilitation of the voice is carried out in relation to the needs of the whole person. This will be dealt with when discussing management of adult voice disorders later. Stemple (1984) points out that individuals who have become aware of their voice difficulties tend to feel that they are saving their voices if they consciously lower the pitch they use. This, in effect, is a misuse of the vocal properties that tax the muscular system, thus accelerating the laryngeal fatigue. Direct pitch modification is in order where this is the case.

Other approaches

In 1952 Froeschels described the *chewing method*. Froeschels started from the premise that as chewing and speech use the same muscles, proper muscular balance for speech could be restored by extending the natural balance of chewing. The stages in this therapy are:

1. chewing breath is substituted for speaking;
2. practise silent, vigorous chewing using a wide variety of chewing postures;
3. add phonation to the chewing practice;
4. intersperse words into the chewing;
5. alternate chewing and talking, then reading and conversation;
6. fade chewing motions leaving naturally balanced phonation.

This holistic approach is particularly appropriate for children. Adults may resist it as it embarrasses them. Perkins (1977) states that treatment begins by emitting and identifying the 'feel' of the vocal elements of optimally balanced voice. He continues:

> How the voice feels provides much more certain guidance for its production than feedback of how it sounds. Listening to one's own voice can be misleading; a speaker can approach 'objective' guidance of phonation better by feel than by ear.
>
> (p. 396)

He also mentions an important point when he says that because the voice tires, especially in later therapy when louder tones may be used, short, frequent practice periods not in excess of 5 minutes should be used.

The Boone Voice Program for Children, the rationale of which is based on Boone's book *The Voice and Voice Therapy*, aims to assess, evaluate and remediate dysphonia in children. Management follows a comprehensive voice rating exercise which includes testing pitch, loudness, quality, nasal resonance, oral resonance, rate and range. The rate of diadochokinesis is measured and an oral mechanism examination is carried out. Following this investigation a programme is designed to meet each individual child's needs.

On the whole, voice disorders are relatively rare in children, and the most common are usually of short duration.

SELECTIVE MUTISM

The terms 'selective' and 'elective' are both employed when discussing this condition. *Selective* will be used here. Technically this is not a true speech disorder. In most cases there is a psychological factor which inhibits the use of speech in particular circumstances. However, it should be mentioned in this context as teachers, carers and, on rare occasions, parents may refer such a child for speech therapy. In 1975, a survey was made in Birmingham which found a prevalence of selective mutism in 7.2 per 1000 schoolchildren during their first school term (Brown and Lloyd, 1975). They reported a gradual diminution of the muteness until by the fifth term of schooling only one child was totally mute. After studying some of the family characteristics of the children involved, and comparing them with matched controls, Brown and Lloyd disclosed the following findings:

1. a positive correlation between mutism and large families;
2. child not usually the firstborn;
3. at least one parent found to be shy;
4. equal distribution of boys and girls;
5. majority of the children were shy and timid;
6. higher incidence found in children of ethnic families, usually with non-English speaking mothers.

Children with selective mutism (SM) have been treated by several professionals including teachers, speech therapists, psychiatrists and psychologists. Sluckin (1977), a senior psychiatric social worker, describes two cases whom she treated successfully using behaviour modification. The treatment extended over five months in one case and over two school terms in the other and involved family, teachers, headteacher and children at school. Both children described presented with most of the characteristics described above. In the first instance, much of the therapy was carried out at home, and consisted mostly of the social worker helping the boy with his reading. Eventually, by means of a tape recorder in the staff room, the head- and class-teachers listened to a tape of the boy reading, in his presence. Finally, the boy agreed to read in the classroom in the presence of another boy. Gradually more children joined the group until, with much help and encouragement, the boy was able to operate normally at school. The second case followed similar lines with most of the work being done during weekly visits by the social worker to the school. Behavioural modification was used in both cases. All verbal responses were rewarded by sweets and praise.

Kolvin and Fundudis (1981) make a distinction between traumatic mutism, in which use of speech ceases totally, and SM where speech is confined to intimates only. The former is a rare condition. SM is reported in some children with normal, age-appropriate speech development who appear to become fixated at the stage of extreme shyness which usually ceases after 3;0. It seems likely that SM occurs in children predisposed to *mild* speech/language disorders who encounter environmental problems which they find difficult to cope with. For example, it has been mooted that the effect of persistent shallow breathing on voice projection may be associated with SM.

Children with SM are often from minority groups on the fringe of society. Reed (1963) suggested that SM may be a learned pattern of behaviour. This possibility could well explain some of the unusual factors surrounding the child and her/his situation in society. Cunningham *et al.* (1983) treated cases by 'shaping', 'situation fading' and 'individual fading'. Thus the treatment of SM is more within the remit of psychologists and behaviour therapists than that of speech therapists.

Sluckin *et al.* (1990) record that there is a higher ratio of girls to boys than in most speech/language disorders, and where there is normal intelligence the prognosis is good. Maturation accounts for improvement in some instances. They have found a high incidence of family psychopathology in families of children with SM.

Several cases with this condition have been treated, a few unsuccessfully, but in most the prognosis is favourable.

7

Adult speech

Adult speech production may be viewed from four aspects: normal; disordered due to continuation of a basic developmental disorder; disordered due to acquired disease or trauma; effects of the ageing process.

NORMAL DEVELOPMENT

It should be remembered that language and speech develop through succeeding developmental stages from birth to death. The infant has to develop towards a state of readiness for using speech, and thence through several stages of development until she/he is equipped to produce acceptable speech as similar to that of the adult model as is possible to attain. This statement assumes a degree of perfection in all that is adult. Of course, this is far from the case. Adult speech, like every other aspect of 'adultness' is dependent on the individual genotype of each person and is subject to innumerable physical and environmental variations. The stages through which the individual passes extend from infancy through childhood to young adulthood, which lasts until about 35 years of age. These are the prime years for speech production as for all other skills. Middle age follows and lasts until about 60 years after which the person is considered elderly. The final stage is old age which terminates in death.

Each individual has his/her inherited strengths and weaknesses in the form of predispositions. These take many guises. One weakness, for example, which occurs fairly frequently, affects the production of voice which in turn, affects the production of speech. People predisposed to dysphonia – 'losing one's voice' –

each time they catch cold, have a specific problem with speech production. (Other people may either have a chest or nasal weakness which is always affected by colds.) As described in the case of children with a similar predisposition, care has to be taken to avoid vocal abuse and misuse in such circumstances, as this can result in the growth of vocal nodules or other unwelcome forms of neoplasms such as ulcers. It is sometimes thought that lack of care in this type of case may encourage cancerous growths but there is no firm evidence for this assumption. A percentage of speakers in each age group will manifest this particular weakness. Some will suffer from psychogenic voice disorders of a similar nature.

Experience has shown that it is no longer possible to divorce the brain and the 'mind'. The existence of the latter appears to result from the normal integration and function of the former. The two are inter-dependent. Blakemore (1988) states that the 'mind' is a product of the brain. Areas within the brain have been identified as centres of emotion. This being the case, it has to be accepted that disturbances at emotional levels in subjects predisposed to some laryngeal/pharyngeal weakness will also disrupt such aspects as the onset and maintenance of voice. This type of vocal strain is likely to result from 'stress'. The latter is one of the penalties of modern competitive working and living and can be extremely difficult to eradicate. Where the inherited weakness applies to the vocal folds, dysphonia will result. Whenever the vicissitudes of life appear to be unbearable, such individuals will manifest a diminution or loss of voice. The balance of resonance will also be affected.

The acquisition of the skill of motor implementation appears to continue into early adolescence (Netsell, 1986) He claims that the adult system represents the developmental continuum and, 'as such, reflects the elegance to which the developing system aspires and can be compared' (p. 3). A further observation by Netsell of considerable interest is that not only is the larynx a source of sound for voicing and a frequency generator for pitch, but also, certain laryngeal muscles can be regarded in their concerted action as an articulator in the same way as tongue, lips and velopharynx. Thus, the coordinative role of the vocal folds with the lips and other structures becomes critical as reflected in the voice onset time (VOT) measure. Kent (1976) indicated that the VOT does not reach adult-like precision until around 11 years of age.

The complete control of speech production is dependent on an extensive system serving the 'final motor pathway for speech', Broca's area, in the frontal lobe of the left hemisphere of the brain. This is influenced by strong subcortical connections, e.g. limbic-frontal-Broca in the precentral region with separate inputs to the basal ganglia and, via the pontine nuclei, to the cerebellum. Speech is goal-directed and afferent-guided. It meets the general motor requirements of a fine motor skill. Wolff (1979) enumerated these requirements. Speech:

1. is performed with accuracy and speed;
2. uses knowledge of results;
3. is improved by practice;
4. demonstrates motor flexibility in achieving goals;
5. relegates all of this to automatic control, where 'consciousness' is freed from the details of action plans.

CONTINUING DEVELOPMENTAL DISORDERS

Disorders of development, such as those already described with reference to childhood disorders, may be perpetuated into adulthood if they are of greater than moderate severity. For example, relatively severe structural deviations which have been either untreated or which have not responded to intervention may persist throughout life and may result in permanently disrupted speech production. Similarly, disorders ensuing from defective or markedly immature cerebral growth and/or functioning will continue to interfere with or retard the complete acquisition of speech. In other words, the production of speech will not be commensurate with the individual's chronological age. Therapeutic intervention may be necessary throughout the greater part of life in such circumstances.

Disorders of fluency such as stuttering and cluttering are latently present within the individual as part of her/his make-up. Cluttering will be apparent in all his/her behaviours, particularly in the speed of delivery, and to varying degrees according to the individual, in different aspects of prosody, articulation and phonation. Cluttering will persist throughout life. Stuttering is liable to reappear when stressful circumstances arise all through the individual's life.

Those may take the form of illness, emotional adjustments, changes of employment and other related deviations from normal routine. Most adults who stutter have been able to reach a level of speech competence through either the support of good intervention, strategies worked out by themselves or, most often, a measure of both. Claims are made by different experts that certain treatment approaches are most successful. It is probably fortunate that so many techniques of management are available as there seems to be the need for numerous idiosyncratic approaches from individual to individual. Reference will be made to a few of these techniques in the section on adult management (p. 119).

ACQUIRED DISORDERS DUE TO DISEASE OR TRAUMA

Dysarthrias

These factors in adolescence and adulthood account for several breakdowns in the production of speech. The most common result of acquired breakdown is some form of dysarthria. Discussion has already taken place regarding the forms of dysarthria affecting child speech (Chapter 3, pp. 36–7). Several disease-specific conditions should be considered which may cause dysarthria in adults. For example, people with *Parkinson's disease* display apparent heterogeneity in both limb problems and speech disorders. Frequently, reduced loudness and a unique voice quality is present. Variations in speed of production occur, some very slow and some much quicker than normal. Many have difficulty in initiating speech while often there is a marked fluctuation in intelligibility. Although it seems likely that rigidity can become uneven in the facial muscles there is still no firm evidence of this. However, it has been noted that the range and velocity of lower lip movement may be more reduced than upper lip movement in some individuals. Continuing research should assist those attempting to alleviate the problems arising, but there can be so many individual variations in the motor behaviour observed that assessment will always need to be carried out in great detail.

Other neurological disorders affecting adults and resulting in dysarthrias include *pseudobulbar palsy*, *motor neurone disease*, *myasthenia gravis*, *Bell's palsy*, *polyneuritis* and *neoplasms*. Pseudobulbar palsy usually results from the occurrence of 'stroke' illness affecting first one hemisphere, followed by a further episode affecting the opposite hemisphere, that is, usually on at least one occasion the patient may have suffered transient dysphasia of one form or another. This is often apparently totally resolved before the onset of dysarthria.

Adolescents will also suffer from dysarthrias in cases of *muscular dystrophy* and other similar genetically based diseases.

A disease which can radically change speech production is cancer. Depending on the site and type of the neoplasm there is the possibility of several examples of disordered articulation and resonance. Dysarthria can occur where space-filling growths invade the brain.

Trauma, such as that caused by *road traffic accidents* (RTAs), frequently leaves victims affected with dysarthria. This is often due to the 'shunt' effect on the brain (where a sharp blow to the front of head leads to violent backward movement of the brain within the skull to the extent that there is damage to the occipital-cerebral and cerebellar regions from the impact). This creates circumstances in which speech production may be severely affected. Sporting accidents can be instrumental in causing problems in producing speech. For example in boxing, brain damage may result in dysarthria, while blows to the face can cause deflection of the nasal septum, depression of the nostrils, contusions to the lips and cheeks and fractures to the bones, all of which may lead to distorted speech and resonance production. Those are some of the external causes of abnormal speech, which could be viewed as self-induced.

Increasingly, it is becoming apparent that habitual practices such as drug-taking, glue sniffing and excessive alcohol, also in the category of self-induced conditions, produce dysarthric symptoms. The side-effects of some types of medication include the development of dysarthria. In all of those cases where intake of some form of unacceptable substance produces muscle weakness, nothing can be done until the habit factor has been tackled and the practice broken. If this is left for too long, complete recovery is not always possible.

Treatment is similar to that previously described for use with children with developmental dysarthria. Emphasis should always be placed on tailoring every management plan to the needs of each individual.

Disorders of phonation

Endocrinological

These are probably the next most frequent problems of production after dysarthrias to which both young and older adults are prone. A small number of developing males do not proceed normally through the process of vocal fold growth and succeeding voice deepening which takes place during the middle teens. Greene (1980) calls this failure of the adolescent male voice to break 'puberphonia'. In the US the terms 'mutational voice disorder' and 'mutational falsetto' are used. This process is dependent upon the hormonal changes which finally determine individual aspects of adulthood. Again there are innumerable variables from person to person, most of which are inherited. Extreme forms of this condition result in syndromes such as Klinefelter's which is X-linked and in which signs include:

1. gross motor delay in childhood;
2. usually normal intelligence but sometimes mental handicap;
3. distractable and occasionally withdrawn as children;
4. delayed emotional maturity and stability;
5. scant facial expression;
6. late onset and progress of puberty;
7. presence of female characteristics particularly a high pitched voice.

All of those features may be present to a reduced extent in mild cases and the most noticeable sign may be the voice pitch which may lead to embarrassment for both the individual and those around him. Occasionally normal voice quality develops in late teenage. It was previously believed that this condition was always psychogenic, but it is now accepted that there are variations of endocrine secretions in each individual which determine the degree of hormonal balance and produce more or fewer sexual characteristics.

Sometimes, in males with normal vocal fold growth, a psychogenic condition arises which results in the use of a falsetto voice. This can often be traced to a desire to perpetuate, or return to, a state of childhood and its attendant protective attributes. Luchsinger and Arnold (1965) refer to a possible organic basis for persistence of childish vocal habits and immaturity in some young men. The fact that some adolescents reject the idea of adulthood and wish to retain strong relationships with their mothers may also influence their vocal use. The only child seems to be more prone to the latter type of vocal anomaly.

Conversely, reports are available of females displaying male qualities of voice. Luchsinger and Arnold (1965) mention cases of schizophrenic women who, among other male characteristics, presented with low male voices, some even described as baritone in quality. Those writers claimed that such virilization of the voice appears to be due to increased activity of the adrenal cortex, causing inhibition of the gonads and inversion of the secondary sex characteristics.

Finally, it should be noted that there is a tendency for some women to suffer some degree of voice disorder associated with sex gland changes and development. Several women evince huskiness during menstruation, due to endocrine imbalance creating a slight oedema at this time. They may also have reduced muscle tone and pitch limitations for the same reason. Changing sexual habits and/or partners may require physical adjustment for such individuals and dysphonia may be a symptom during the transition period. The presence of other endocrine imbalance(s) may disrupt the normal activities of the sex hormones and produce side-effects requiring treatment. Dysphonia may become an unwelcome problem during the period of menopause or following surgery for hysterectomy. This is most likely to occur in those women who have had a tendency to some dysphonia before and during menstruation, that is, whose vocal mechanisms have been predisposed to some degree (it may only have been a mild degree) of reflected weakness throughout life.

Treatment for such voice changes includes the use of hormones (hormone replacement therapy) in an attempt to achieve a healthy balance. This is not always a successful form of treatment as undesirable side-effects may result. Often women of this age have to contend with numerous irritating little changes which disrupt their comfort and undermine their confidence. Counselling the immediate family is frequently an important part of therapy. In addition, basic treatment to ascertain the fundamental frequency, the correct pitch, rate and stress patterns required for the best sound production and awareness of breathing and relaxation techniques are still the most important factors on which to build treatment.

Until recently, excessive smoking often aggravated dysphonia in the menopausal years. There is less smoking nowadays and many women have only mild symptoms where previously they would have had much greater problems. Heavy drinking may have a similar effect causing more severe dysphonic problems. The results of both of those habits are chronic laryngitis, cough and a marked lowering of pitch. Cutting down, or preferably cutting out, smoking and heavy drinking will considerably improve the situation.

Management of all conditions which arise from imbalance of hormones is a completely medical matter dependent on the administration of the necessary medication to redress the balance. Thus, the role of the speech therapist is one of referral to the appropriate agency. However, it is important for the clinician to be familiar with the various symptoms which can occur in such circumstances. Frequently, however, the consultant will re-refer the patient to the speech therapist to apply the finishing-off techniques. This occurs due to the prevalence of counter-productive habits which have been acquired over the years. The layman is often unaware of the production of speech and even the simplest explanation may be sufficient to establish new and better habits which will remove the strains which have been adversely affecting vocal production in the past.

Other endocrine imbalances may lead to voice disorders. For example, decreased or increased thyroid hormone will affect voice production. Before the use of thyroxin in cases where there was a marked decrease in the release of thyroid hormones, *cretinism* was a relatively common occurrence. As well as reduced growth in limb and general body size, this condition interfered with laryngeal and therefore vocal fold growth. The voice qualities which resulted included huskiness, weakness and soft breathy vocal attack. The vocal range was small and the pitch high and monotonous. Fortunately, cretinism is rarely found in Western countries nowadays, due to screening at birth.

Older children and adults may, however, still develop *myxoedema* which is a constitutional disorder due to decrease or absence of thyroid hormones. Such decreased production of those hormones may result from atrophy or removal of the thyroid gland, reduction or lack of normal pituitary stimulation or following the use of drugs. The major vocal symptom is hoarseness, which, in turn, is derived from the wasting of the laryngeal muscles. Laryngoscopy may reveal bowing of the vocal folds which is recognized as a further result of muscular atrophy and which

105

in itself is responsible for the hoarse, weakened and excessively low voice production. Alternatively, where there is an increased flow of hormones from the thyroid gland, different forms of hyperthyroidism will develop, producing a different type of hoarseness, usually displaying breathiness with reduced volume. *Thyrotoxicosis* is possibly the most common condition in which dysphonia associated with hyperthyroidism is found. This is characterized chiefly by increased frequency of respiration and reduced vital capacity. These breathing disorders may be complicated by emotional instability presenting as inexplicable anxiety, nervous excessive irritability and frequent bouts of exhaustion.

A few cases have been reported of dysphonia due to hyperparathyroidism (Simpson, 1954). This may have arisen from an imbalance of calcium and phosphorus metabolism. It is known that the parathyroid has a part to play in the regulation of those metabolisms. Overexcitability of the muscles can follow even a slight decrease of ionized calcium in the blood serum and the opposite effect would result from an increased blood calcium level. Both of those irregularities could cause dysphonia.

Some diseases may upset the functioning of the adrenal glands and in cases of both hypo- and hyper-adrenalism the action of the laryngeal muscles will be affected. Similarly, disease or damage to the pituitary gland will be reflected in the activity of the vocal folds. The major function of the pituitary gland is the regulation of body growth. Either too much or too little growth will produce some disorder of the voice.

Disease

When cancer attacks parts of the vocal tract, different surgical intervention may be necessary. Morrish (1988) reports a case of total glossectomy in which, despite the fact that the whole tongue had to be removed, the client was able to produce adequate and recognizable articulatory patterns, from the viewpoints of both the speaker and the listener.

Probably the most dramatic and therefore the most documented result of cancer occurs when the larynx is involved. In their unique position within the 'bony' fortress provided by the shape and structure of the larynx, the vocal folds are well protected. (The larynx is, of course, cartillaginous, not bony.) Carcinomic cells can and do invade this area in varying forms. In cases where the neoplasm is completely contained within the larynx and where radiotherapy has failed to kill the invading cells and stop further growth, it is necessary to make surgical intervention to remove the whole larynx. This step usually rids the individual of the cancer and many years of healthy life may follow. If the neoplastic cells have extended into the pharyngeal and/or oesophageal areas the prognosis is less good. Alternatively, there are occasions when hemilaryngectomy or supraglottic laryngectomy may be required. Since the initial, and probably the major, function of the larynx is to act as a valve to protect the tracheae and lungs from the aspiration of swallowed liquids and solids, redirection of organs is required following total laryngectomy. Direct oral breathing cannot continue through the mouth so the trachea is redirected, sutured to the neck and a stoma, or hole, is created through which vital breathing can take place. This necessitates the acquisition of a second, controlled breathing system with which to produce speech. Many older or less able patients find this difficult. The passage of food and drink remains the same after surgery. Vocal rehabilitation is essential after all these operations.

The Ageing Process

Possibly the most important aspect about vocal changes observed in elderly and old subjects is that they influence listeners' perceptions regarding the age of the speaker. Morris and Brown (1987) report a study in which two groups of healthy women, 25 aged 20–35 and 25 over 75 years of age, were tested by several procedures to determine whether age-related differences in speech and voice exist between populations of old and younger speakers. The younger group were considered to be typical of their age range. The older women were selected for their independence, capability and possession of hearing acuity within normal limits. Intensity procedures, air pressure and phoneme duration procedures were used with both groups. Results indicated that vocal effort by the elderly, at conversational levels, is not significantly altered by the ageing process. In studies of the male voice, different researchers found different variations in several vocal characteristics. Those included voice tremor, imprecise consonants, laryngeal tension, low pitch and hoarseness. Thus it can be seen that the production of speech becomes affected in some older people to some degree.

A specific condition which is found in a number of relatively

107

young adults and people with Down's syndrome around 40 years of age, also, and more frequently, affects older people of over 60;0. This is Alzheimer's disease. A considerable amount of research is taking place to try to understand the many variables which constitute this condition. One of the areas least affected is articulation. Often the physical problems of Alzheimer sufferers are minimal, but sensory awareness deteriorates and overall appropriateness decreases. Thus the problem is one of language rather than speech or voice.

With age, deterioration in muscle strength, control and consistency occurs which may affect movements and result in a reduction of clarity, speed and effective production. Intelligibility suffers in such circumstances. Hearing also deteriorates with the passage of time interfering with self-monitoring. Although this is most likely to disrupt the comprehension and appropriateness of language, it may also precede a lowering of articulatory and resonance ability. Despite the fact that there is a general decline in sensory and motor performance as an inevitable consequence of ageing, there is a marked difference in the rate and extent of such decline. Extreme individual variation in the deterioration of motor performance is one of the most robust findings in ageing research (Spirduso, 1982).

Articulation appears to be less affected by ageing than voice production. Ryan and Burk (1974) suggested that the vocal tremor, laryngeal tension, air loss, imprecise consonants and low rate of articulation noted in the speech of the aged may reflect that these speakers are at the mild end of a continuum of dysarthria. More recently, Ramig and Ringel (1983) hypothesized that because physiological ageing may not parallel chronological ageing, the physiological condition may be an important variable in the study of the ageing voice. It seems likely that if research were done into cognitive ageing of individuals, this too would be a significant factor in the effect of the ageing process, as attitude, interest and personal resources also help to determine the use and maintenance of the physiological system. Another crucial factor which exerts considerable influence on the whole situation is personality.

Ramig (1986) produces data which suggests that acoustic correlates of degenerative changes include the interactive roles of physiological and functional adjustments to the communication process and must be considered in future research in order to interpret changes in speech with advancing age.

8

Management of adult speech disorders I

Management of adolescent and adult problems will be considered, in the two final chapters, within the categories:

1. normal development;
2. continuation of disordered development;
3. acquired disorders due to disease or trauma;
4. ageing.

NORMAL DEVELOPMENT

Occasional maintenance is required in speakers who for the most part can be regarded as normal. For example, in instances of the insertion of dental prosthesis, even capping of teeth, slight oral-spatial adaptations have to be made. This is usually a matter of trajectory for the tongue, which is quickly mastered. The loss of sensation experienced following injections for dental fillings and extractions helps the healthy adult to appreciate the disadvantages of people with permanent oral, and other, sensory losses. However, as the effects of the medication wear off so do the memories of the inconvenience. Such minor changes do not require intervention. Similarly, injuries to other areas of the vocal tract, resulting in inflammation and swelling, clear up quickly, for the most part, and the slight modifications needed during the period of recovery are short-lived. Likewise, where mild dysarthria occurs due to medication or alcohol, the duration of the disrupted production of articulatory patterns is short term and normal articulatory practices are soon restored. Occasionally, normal adults have brief bouts of dysfluency, possibly due to minimal transient changes in brain function. They pass quickly, leave no apparent trace of change and are forgotten.

People who once or twice a year in the course of a common cold, or once or twice in a lifetime at periods of great stress such as loss or bereavement, 'lose their voices' were previously recommended to undertake 'vocal rest'. This, in fact, means using the voice as little as possible to allow the inflamed tissues to recover. Adults are better able to do this successfully than are children. Once having felt the benefit of the reduction in phonation, adults are also able to implement the practice on further occasions when the need arises. Singers, actors, lecturers, teachers and other habitual voice users may have to consider such rest at various periods throughout their professional careers. It is the basis of recuperation for most vocal problems in the opinion of some clinicians, although others have discontinued its use on the basis that it is old fashioned. Experience indicates that, in association with good breathing habits and general and differential relaxation, this is a reliable and successful approach.

Martin (1988) uses humour and disbelief to compare someone with a bad leg running in a marathon after getting 'something to rub on', with a patient with a bad voice purchasing 'something to gargle', then giving a speech and being unable to understand why this led to complete loss of voice. Distortions of voice as well as other disruptions of speech and language may result from the use of some drugs. For example, Gates and Montalbo (1987) report that beta blockers prescribed in high doses to reduce performance anxiety may have a detrimental effect on singing quality. They also indicate that the use of throat sprays may reduce pain or soreness but dampen kinaesthetic feedback so that further damage occurs. Hoarseness has been found as a result of the intake of anti-depressants and also in alcoholics. These and allied factors associated with medication have to be considered by the speech therapist when differential diagnosis is being determined.

In the normal course of events, when women reach menopause some may have to resort to altering or modifying their vocal use. In both situations and in other associated conditions, breathing habits should be observed and measured and adjustments made to facilitate correct breathing. The majority of people do not know, and do not need to know, how they breathe as the mode they adopt seems to serve them satisfactorily throughout life. In the case of disorder this becomes a requirement and better breathing practices may need to be adopted (Appendix A). Also, relaxation therapy may have to be undertaken to ensure even more release from the muscular tensions which often affect the action and movement of the vocal folds (Appendix C).

CONTINUATION OF DISORDERED DEVELOPMENT

When children who have had speech disorders reach adulthood, the majority have acquired a state of competence. Sometimes slight difficulties persist, for example, in the presence of mild dysarthria, mild dyspraxia, mild nasality, lateral sibilants, continuing tendency to thrust the tongue. Most of these conditions are very slight and therefore acceptable. When such persisting characteristics are moderate or severe, they continue to be disabling factors and exclude their users from much of normal social life. For example, Down's syndrome adults will still present with dysarthria to varying degrees of severity. The few adults with developmental articulatory dyspraxia will continue to have problems of intelligibility which will prevent their listeners from understanding their production of speech. Such cases are often considered to have reached their potential and treatment is discontinued. Recent experience shows that human development continues throughout life. Although there will always be a degree of damage which is irremediable, associated development may be taking place and assessments for attainment issuing from this development should be on-going. For example, people who have experienced severe immature articulatory praxis may eventually develop to a stage in later life at which they acquire normal articulatory abilities. Compensatory techniques which were beyond reach at an earlier stage may now be possible.

A different view of speech disorders is usually taken by adolescents than that held by them as children. Parents, teachers and other interested adults have previously 'spoken for them', thus supplying the interventions considered necessary to satisfy the listener. With maturity, the problem becomes one of personal choice and need. This means that self-referrals are made when the difficulty precludes the client from social, occupational and other goals. A more definite and determined emphasis is placed on cooperation and self-improvement. Often, objectives are met relatively quickly, even when as in some cases, they are similar to those set at an earlier stage but not then achieved for lack of motivation and therefore application. Another barrier to competence at this stage in life is the habit factor. This is frequently so strong that not only has the process of production to be changed due to some innate weakness or environmental factor, but the speech forms wrongly adopted have become so set that two layers of production patterns have to be eliminated before successful speech use can be reached. Similar circumstances may arise from institutionalization. Fortunately, these are of rare occurrence.

Stutterers, as well as those with articulation disorders, often refer themselves for another infusion of treatment before an important job interview, or to gain entry into a specific adult group which may require some ability to account for oneself orally. Adults with some form of speech difficulty elect for themselves whether or not to remedy the situation.

Mental handicap

Adults with mental handicap continue to have decisions made for them except in rare cases where they become aware of their personal needs and decide to seek help. People with mental handicap being returned to the community under the present 'normalization' policy should continue to be assessed for language and speech development and/or improvement or deterioration. The extended environmental and peer-group experience which results from sharing life in a house or flat with a small number of people, should be directed in the most beneficial way to encourage integration and independence for each individual. Most of these people are unprepared for such radical upheavals in their lives and it seems inevitable that a great many opportunities will be lost unless speech therapists and other professionals take advantage of these circumstances and provide both suitable therapy and valuable team membership. Lifestyles are changing and with them the need for the greatest possible communicative interactions and practical involvements. Examples in this context would be moderating the volume of utterance for social purposes, and practising turn-taking within the group. These both require pragmatic approaches to the use of speech and language, and motor control as well as cognitive awareness.

Where there are more severe difficulties and people have to be maintained in hospital the debate continues about the value of continued management. It is necessary, however, to maintain a watching brief on such cases to determine the effects of development. Part of the debate itself is the question of whether environment has much influence on development. Does the fact of virtual incarceration, as in long-term hospitalization and the inevitable institutionalization that results, itself detracts from the possibility of acquiring more skills through greater experience? How many of these patients are mentally ill as well as mentally handicapped? Ineichen (1984) reports that probably 50% of the population of a hospital for people with mental handicap pose management problems due to psychiatric disorders. Alternatively, Bicknell (1983) asserts that among people with mental handicap living at home 'only a small proportion suffer from pathological stress, mental illness or behaviour disorder for which psychiatric treatment is relevant'. It is difficult to establish a true picture. Ineichen states that:

> The best way to reduce mental illness and behaviour problems among mentally handicapped people is to remove the conditions that do so much to bring them about. This means providing above all the opportunities for ordinary living that non-handicapped people take for granted.

> (p. 764)

'Normalization' has occurred since Ineichen wrote these words. But lack of resources, both financial and qualitative, with respect to understanding how such people function and what their immediate needs are, has meant that the best possible living conditions have not been created. Often, this results from a communication breakdown of another kind. Planners construct the smaller, home environments on the basis of the needs and comforts of the mentally able, whereas more specific needs may be required for low-achievers who view life differently. Nevertheless, the foundations have been laid for a better future for this population.

Caldwell (personal communication) has refuted, once and for all, the belief that nothing can be done for some of the people in hospitals with severe mental handicaps complicated by unacceptable and antisocial behaviours. However, the method she employs is expensive in money, staff, time and patience. With the cooperation of a clinical psychologist and a research student, Caldwell set up an experiment in a hospital ward devoted to the care of a male clientele who were both profoundly handicapped and disturbed. The focus of the intervention was to design individually

113

appropriate pieces of equipment based on observations made of each client's behaviour, physical disabilities and the knowledge of how developing children learn to manipulate their environment.

The implementation of the programme depended on one-to-one relationships and the willingness of the staff involved to make an objective, in-depth assessment of each person's needs and reactions. The factors considered were personal comfort, identification of secure areas selected by each client, postural preferences (standing, sitting, lying), tolerance to change of environment, presence of obsessional behaviour and identification of possible reinforcers. The materials constructed had to meet needs like left-handedness, inability to extend digital and manual muscles fully and other idiosyncratic traits noted during the preparatory period of observation. Only blue and yellow equipment was made to obviate the presence of colour blindness. Each piece was strongly put together, both to withstand excessive handling and to provide a strong proprioceptive and tactile feedback. Visual and auditory prompts and signals were incorporated where appropriate, and as many perceptual levels were stimulated as possible, without overloading and confusing.

Results were achieved in most cases over short or extended periods. By the end of a year, men who had previously failed to access any means by which they could participate in activities approaching a normal lifestyle were able to interact and communicate in a fashion acceptable in most circumstances. Some made remarkable improvements while others achieved only a small amount, but the benefit to the whole group was significant. In a few cases this progress facilitated the readiness to develop language and speech to some degree and made it possible for the interchange of communication to take place.

As already stated however, the drain, particularly on manpower, is considerable, and society has not yet reached a level at which the financial provision for such involvement is acceptable. In addition, if more individual attention could be given to people with mental handicap of a less severe nature, it is obvious that much more improvement could be expected. Those with severe handicaps could be helped at an earlier stage before behaviour becomes disordered. Agreement about the need to enable all human beings to reach their potential would revolutionize the whole state of the human condition. At present general lack of knowledge of mental handicap and its causes, attitudes towards the subject and lack of resources prevent many governments from even considering such advances, viz. the TV film of the Greek island on which people with mental handicaps are incarcerated, *Horizon* BBC 2, (1990).

Blindness and partial sightedness

Another condition which has an on-going effect on speech development is found in adults who have always been blind. Their need to compensate for loss of sight and therefore loss of experience of non-verbal communication often leaves them with incomplete speech practice. As infants, babbling appears in their development at the normal time, but stops occasionally to give way to listening, and therefore less sound-making is used. Language is also reduced by the inability to experience concepts, e.g. behind, in front of. Word action concepts are difficult to imagine, for example, individuals in different roles such as in sewing, painting, dancing. Also comparing objects in different positions, e.g. on the windowsill in the sunshine, on the shelf in a darkened cupboard.

Blind children appear to use social phrases before naming objects. Their priorities are so different that they may not derive as much pleasure from experimental soundmaking as do sighted children, and so provide for themselves less opportunity for motor practice and thus clearer intelligibility. Also, they may listen more for word meaning than for the prosodic features which enhance meaning, and so fail to produce the interest in speech production provided by intonation, rate, stress and other non-segmental factors. These practices become habitual and may be discernible throughout life.

On the other hand, claims are made that imitation is more prevalent in blind children, possibly due to over-encouragement, so perhaps this balances out the reduction of sound play. Concepts such as colour, tidal movements, facial expression, are unknown quantities, so descriptive words used with those categories may be absent from their vocabularies. Where there is a language/speech problem in addition to the visual one, special techniques have to be used to enable therapy to be carried out. As with the rest of the population, different approaches should be made to individual blind people. For the less sophisticated, one should present oneself by touch, whereas voice would be the means to approach the more sophisticated. Touch is more adaptable however, and can successfully convey tolerance, affection, impatience and many other abstract feelings. A multisensory approach should be aimed for, to share the greatest amount of experience.

It is important to remember when working with people who are not blind but partially sighted that both positioning, and the fact that they may vary the use of vision in different environments, should be carefully considered. To supply the greatest amount of help in a clinical situation, maximum use of their limited sightedness should be made possible.

Voice disorders

No attempts at management for voice disorders should ever be undertaken until a full examination by an Ear, Nose and Throat consultant has taken place to eliminate the possibility of an organic condition which may require medical or surgical intervention. In cases of dysphonia, ill-advised or contrary intervention by the speech therapist can cause actual physical damage. This should never be allowed to occur. Bearing in mind the fact that vocal strain can lead to vocal misuse, which may then result in vocal nodules or vocal ulcers, care must be taken to continue the use of treatment methods appropriate to the needs of the individual with this predisposition.

Andrews *et al.* (1986) describe the comparison of two treatment programmes applied to adults with hyperfunctional voice disorders. There is no indication that any of them were subject to long-term vocal difficulties, but the findings are noteworthy. Five of a group of ten were treated by The Progressive Relaxation Method (PRM) devised by Bernstein and Borkovec (1973) which is based on the work of Jacobson (1938). The remaining five were submitted to the Electromyogram Biofeedback (EMG) programme. The differences in the two programmes were found only in the method of inducing relaxation of the laryngeal musculature.

The PRM relied on making the subjects aware of tension followed by relaxation in groups of muscles. In addition, it incorporated the concept of a calm, mental attitude advocated by several workers, and self-relaxation first proposed by Schultz and Luthe (1959). Training progressed gradually from 16 → 7 → 4 muscle groups and finally to self-relaxation by recall, where all the muscles are relaxed simultaneously. For the experiment, Andrews *et al.* (1986) modified the programme by re-ordering of the muscle groups to progress from the limbs to the finer musculature of the face and the tongue. Tension contrast was removed as soon as relaxation from rest could be achieved successfully, and inclusion of visualization of a calm scene was used as in the autogenic techniques of Schultz and Luthe.

Use of the EMG programme involved visual feedback of laryngeal muscle activity in the form of a needle on a scale, utilized to prevent interference with phonation from an auditory feedback signal. Continuous feedback, recommended by Gaarder and Chase (1971), was employed. Tension reduction trials of one minute duration with a half-minute period between trials were used as indicated by the pilot study. A no-biofeedback trial terminated each stage and each session to ensure that control of laryngeal tension had been consolidated at that level. The other components in both Voice Training Programmes were similar:

relaxation at rest
control of expiration
hum on monotone
extension of pitch range (variety of CV syllables)
extension of phrase length
reading of passage
conversation.

For the purposes of the study the ten subjects were treated as matched pairs. The study revealed that both EMG biofeedback and progressive relaxation succeeded in reducing tension in the laryngeal area and effected improvement in voice quality. At a three month follow-up, improvements in all measures were maintained. Several treatment implications are important as a result of this investigation. Some subjects progressed rapidly on acquisition of the relaxation skill, suggesting that tension was the focal point. Others required a longer period to integrate relaxation with the complex coordination of voice required for connected speech. All subjects benefited from explanations of normal voice and the cause of their dysphonia as recommended by Lerman (1980). Several subjects who had suffered accompanying symptoms such as headaches, sleeping disturbances and neck and shoulder pain reported reductions in all of them. Also, subjects who had been taking painkillers and insomnia drugs indicated a consequent reduction in their doses.

The strategies selected to promote relaxation appeared to be more important than the two methods employed. Relaxation was enjoyed by all the subjects and, with one exception, all commented on increased awareness of daily tension and the ability to reduce it successfully. Once again, the uniqueness of each client was noted and the necessity to consider the psychological, physical and personality factors and their interactions on voice production was emphasized. This calls for open-mindedness, knowledge and competence from clinicians.

Consideration of this type of investigation suggests that for individuals with a tendency to voice disorder, management at the earliest possible stage should include relaxation to the point of self-relaxation. This involves the client taking the decision to self-administer therapy and the clinician taking time to describe the problem, help the client to understand it and to impart the treatment in such a way that s/he may apply it at any time without further recourse to the therapist. However, it should be remembered that the nature of voice disorders indicates that many of them will recur in new, tense or frightening situations and that part of the clients' need seems to be for supportive interaction. In other words, a large part of dysphonia is psychogenic in character.

Differential diagnosis becomes extremely difficult in circumstances where there are coexisting disorders such as dysarthrophonia, in which there are elements of muscle weakness involving not only the muscles of articulation but also those of phonation. Alternatively, psychogenic hoarseness may co-occur with neurological deficit with no relationship to the dysphonia. For example, if an adult with cerebral palsy and the resultant dysarthria has to be hospitalized for surgery for, say, appendicitis, it is possible that he/she may develop a psychogenic dysphonia due to anxiety. The speech therapist may alleviate this condition by manoeuvring the larynx downwards to decrease the effort brought about by increased tension. This minimal repositioning lowers the pitch and reduces strain and hoarseness. An intelligent client will perhaps be able to maintain this improvement if it is accompanied by careful, appropriate counselling.

Greene (1984) describes a study of a small number of clients with functional dysphonia who tended to hyperventilate. Hyperventilation is said to occur when ventilation of the lungs is in excess of metabolic needs. From this limited study it can be concluded that there is a relationship between anxiety and breathing disorder, and this supports the effectiveness of relaxation, breathing training and appropriate counselling as therapy in this type of speech disorder.

Stuttering therapies

As has been previously indicated when discussing management of child stuttering, many approaches exist and most have already been mentioned (pp. 71–80).

Adults who stutter frequently have few problems with speech production in the normal course of events. When difficulties do arise following illness, stress, fatigue or other upsets, self-referral is common and motivation is high. The personal construct theory (Fransella, 1970) has proved successful with certain types of people who stutter and who respond to the repertory grid technique based on the work of Kelly (1955). The ability to come to terms with her/his self-concept and to determine that s/he is an individual who stutters but retains her/his individuality, as opposed to seeing her/himself as part of an amorphous group, 'stutterers', has enabled several people to control and accept their speech difficulties. In some cases, the stuttering has been overcome altogether.

Use of the Monterey programmed stuttering therapy has become popular with some British clinicians. Based on operant conditioning principles, this therapy has met the needs of child, adolescent and adult clients. More research is required to determine long-term results of this treatment, but it seems that the therapy is satisfactory to some degree to both clinicians and clients.

ACQUIRED DISORDERS DUE TO DISEASE OR TRAUMA

A feature of contemporary life is the incidence of road traffic accidents (RTA). Many young men of 16–25 frequently lose their ability to produce acceptable speech due to head injuries contracted by RTA. Motor cyclists outnumber motorists in this context. There are also other types of accident which, as has been mentioned previously, befall young sportspeople including skiing, swimming, boxing, cricket and, in fact, all strenuous games, in which head injuries may be acquired. Speech disorders, primarily dysarthria, may also be an effect of the intake of specific drugs used, albeit illegally, in sporting circles. Management of such conditions is predominantly a team affair with the speech therapist as an important team member. The aim of treatment is a return to normality but frequently irreversible brain damage has resulted and the prognostic outlook may be poor.

Communication treatment is essential at every level as the success of all members of the management team depends on the individual's ability to comprehend, by some means, the instructions and directions of the different professionals involved. (It is also important that communication channels between team members are kept open. It is always worth the speech therapist's time to discuss the mechanics of human communication in normal circumstances with team colleagues at a completely objective level.) Dysarthria and dysphasia-with-dyspraxia often result from the brain damage incurred by the young person involved. A programme to deal with such dysarthria will include:

1. breathing and phonating exercises to correct the damage to muscles and restore a degree of control;
2. feeding exercises to help chewing and swallowing;
3. prosodic exercises to reinstate intonation, exert control over rate, pitch and volume;
4. articulation exercises to improve muscle movement, replace sensory feedback and enhance intelligibility;
5. conversational practice.

The above exercises will be most effective if they are dovetailed into an overall approach which would include physical and occupational therapy. Family and friends should also be involved in the programme as frequently major modifications have to be made in everyday living and the sooner everyone realizes the limitations of the accident victim, the better will be the chances for the future. The majority of people find it difficult to comprehend the fact that all will not return to normal in most of these cases. The burden of a brain-damaged person has to be experienced to be fully appreciated. For the methodology employed in exercises 1–4, see appendices A, D and E. Conversational practice is best carried out by group therapy in which specific, shared subjects are selected for general discussion. Each group member should be counselled regarding the importance of appropriate interaction and inclusion in the exercise.

A similar programme of speech production will be followed by an adult who has dysphasia-with-dypraxia, with the addition of considerable work of a kinaesthetic and proprioceptive nature to stimulate the sense of feeling which will usually be disrupted.

(*Kinaesthesis* is muscle sense, perception of movement; *propri-oception* is sensation from muscles and joints, conveying infor-mation, not always consciously perceived, about their position in relation to the rest of the body so that posture is maintained by reflex movement.) For example, using visual cueing in front of a mirror, start by employing passive movements of the tongue and lips by the clinician. This helps to institute basic kinaesthetic awareness and depends on the laying down of a store of kinaes-thetic memories for skilled actions. After a reasonable time during which these passive movements may be stimulating the desired awareness, encourage the client to move passively his/her own tongue and lips, concentrating on the build-up of feeling which should result. The objective is to bring motor pattern production to surface awareness and control. Now encourage client to make the same movements actively. When this is successful, proceed to repetition of motor sequences and eventually, in severe cases, to emphasis of consonant-vowel (CV) and vowel-consonant (VC) syllables and, in mild cases, to the use of appropriate words and phrases. Several workers advocate the use of strategically placed food or mouthwash to direct tongue and lip movements.

Adults with acquired articulatory dyspraxia may benefit from *Melodic Intonation Therapy (MIT)*. This employs the use of intoned sequences during the formulation of propositional lan-guage. It has been noted that while MIT is directed toward lan-guage, poor articulation has been improved by its adapted use, as well as a reduction in the frequency of phonemic errors (Sparks and Holland, 1976). In addition to intoned sequences, tapping is used in this imitative programme.

There may also be an element of spatial/temporal difficulty resulting from the loss of body image and/or identity in the environment. It is established that human beings need to experi-ence positions for themselves before they can relate them to exter-nal objects. Thus, *inside, outside, in front, behind, underneath* or *on top* have to be worked out with the individual's body as the focal point in the first instance. Once these relationships have been re-established it is then possible to deal with similar relationships outside of the self. Repeated exercises help to facilitate this aware-ness and centre the person's world of movement and action. Tricky features like 'the back of your left knee', 'under your right heel' and other more obscure body parts may have become impossible to retrieve. Such loss of awareness should always be tested for and considered in the management programme. It is acknowledged that a major part of this difficulty may be psycholinguistic as well as moto-spatial.

An additional time lag may be present which means that longer motor processing as well as motor planning time is required and the operation of muscle function may have become unacceptably slow. Sequencing of movements will often have to be worked on, and this of course may affect digital and other muscular movements connected with communication, as well as articulatory movements. A measure of inconsistency may further compound attempts to produce acceptable pronunciation patterns. In such cases it is absolutely essential to devote time to explaining and clarifying the situation to relatives and carers. Often clients are treated, through lack of understanding, as though they have become mentally handicapped and their self-confidence and motivation plummet.

9

Management of adult speech disorders II

Pursuing the management of speech disorders in adults, this chapter is concerned with phonation, resonance and the specific problems of the aged. Disorders of resonance may take one of two forms: hyper- or hyponasality.

HYPERNASALITY

This condition is due to a velopharyngeal insufficiency usually attributable to a structural, muscular or nerve disability in the velopharyngeal area. Nasal sounds, /m/, /n/ and /ŋ/, occur at an average rate of more than one a second in normal speech. Where oral sounds are nasalized, this means that hypernasality is indeed marked and correction is required. Once again, management is highly individualized. Careful assessment is necessary to isolate the specific cause of the problem. Usually the first stage of any treatment involves increasing the efficiency of the velopharyngeal sphincter. This can often be managed by physical means. The habit factor, where present, may become the greatest management problem, and a programme of conscious listening for the purposes of self-monitoring may have to be adopted. Improvement of hypernasality is based on structured voice and speech procedures and selected physical exercise, for example:

1. adequate oral breath pressure;
2. oral air flow and correct breath direction;
3. correct muscular tension;
4. swallowing, sucking, blowing and whistling.

It has been acknowledged that the greatest improvement in communication in individuals with cleft palate comes from improved precision of articulation; this results in better intelligibility and less perceived hypernasality. Tactile, kinaesthetic and visual approaches are superior to using the auditory channel to improve articulation. Listening training techniques are of prime importance in identifying oral-nasal balance.

Stemple (1984) proposes the following 10-step voice therapy outline applied to resonance:

Step 1   clinician explains balanced resonance and its dependence upon an adequate velopharyngeal seal except during the production of the nasal sounds, with the rule being to use correct resonance balance;

Step 2   client uses listening training to discriminate resonance imbalance in others;

Step 3   client uses listening training to discriminate resonance balance in others;

Step 4   client uses listening training to discriminate how resonance imbalance *sounds* and *feels* in himself;

Step 5   client learns resonance control by how his/her voice *sounds* and *feels* when resonance is balanced;

Step 6   client discovers where resonance balance is used;

Step 7   client finds where resonance imbalance is used;

Step 8   use of adequate resonance balance *some* of the time;

Step 9   use of adequate resonance balance *most* of the time;

Step 10 use of adequate resonance balance *all* of the time.

In assessment, consideration should also be given to loudness, pitch and rate to ensure good use of resonance. A programme may have to be planned and implemented to adjust the above features before appropriate use of resonance is achieved. For example, with reference to loudness, voice fading at the end of sentences may have to be elementary. This is achieved by breaking up sentences into phrases, words and syllables and discussing the relevance of emphasizing important parts of the sentence. Pauses may be introduced between parts of the sentence to illustrate the emphasis required. With the emergence of loudness control, sentences can then be practised without the pauses.

Pitch lowering may help a person to make an automatic shift in resonance characteristics in his/her voice. This modification helps to reduce or eliminate hypernasality. As long as the pitch level is kept within the person's optimum range, and the individual is encouraged to start sentences at a lower pitch than that used previously, pitch control will be achieved. This results in decreasing perceived hypernasality.

Workers disagree as to whether rate should be increased or decreased to reduce hypernasality. At present, the tendency is for the rate to be speeded up to attain this goal. Negative practice proves successful towards the end of a programme to achieve a reduction in hypernasality. This enables the client to practise the correct and incorrect forms and to establish firmly the discrimination between the two.

Awareness of the location of tension will also help the client to deal with this problem. For example, clients may substitute a glottal replacement for various pressure sounds. What they appear to be doing is substituting a build-up of pressure at the level of the glottis for a build-up of pressure at the appropriate placement within the oral cavity. Alleviation of this habit can be brought about by listening practice, in which the client listens to become aware of the difference between a glottal stop and the correct production in the clinician's speech. Next, the client has to make the same differentiation in the production of her/his own speech. Where there is some difficulty in the auditory modality, it may be necessary to use visual, proprioceptive and kinaesthetic cues to create the awareness level required. For the correction of hypernasality on vowel sounds Greene (1980) suggested that the teeth should be well separated and the back of the tongue, pillars of fauces and the pharynx should be relaxed.

Cooper (1973) suggests eliminating hypernasality with the use of vowels which stress oral resonance such as /o/ and /u/. Although Cooper uses this method with children it can be modified for adult use. This is the sequence of steps employed:

1. Say /o/ repeatedly, using the lowest level of optimal pitch range until the resonance is acceptable. The clinician is used as the model and supportive audio-recordings are made and evaluated.
2. The process is repeated with /u/.
3. Now follow the vowels with a number – /o/ one, /o/ two /u/ one, /u/ two, counting to ten in this manner.
4. Next combine the vowels and numbers – /o/ /u/ one, /o/ /u/ two, counting to ten. Monitor resonance carefully throughout.

5. Add single words – /o/ /u/ 'one hello', /o/ /u/ 'one house', gradually adding more words – /o/ /u/ 'two tomorrow'.
6. Sentences now follow the production of /o/ /u/ – /o/ /u/ 'one, the sun is setting tomorrow'.
7. Finally, appropriate and balanced oral-nasal resonance is practised in spontaneous speech. These speech samples are audiotaped and monitored to control hypernasality. (Experience shows that this method does not necessarily work for intrapersonal self-monitoring).

Similarly, there is no guarantee that the intrapersonal as well as the interpersonal component of self-monitoring is accounted for.

The *pull-out* exercise can be used when a client is asked to repeat a word such as '*house*' ten times, gradually pulling out of an initial hypernasal quality, until the last few productions are free of hypernasality. Again audiotapes are useful for evaluation. Then the use of voiceless stop consonants, such as /p/ and /t/ initially, are introduced as they require an increase in air pressure in the oral cavity with resulting tight velopharyngeal sphincter closure. Word pairs are also used in this pull-out exercise, such as 'pie-my', 'tip-nip'. With reference to *loudness*, increasing vocal intensity may help to reduce hypernasality, especially for those who habitually talk softly. Increased loudness demands more efficient use of the pharyngeal and oral cavities and so tends to off-set cul-de-sac resonance, as well as improving muscle tone. When this results, through listening practice in improved resonance, therapy can proceed to maintaining good resonance at a reduced loudness level.

There may be less perceived hypernasality at certain voice pitch levels than at others. Saying vowels at various pitch levels may isolate vowels which are free from hypernasality. When non-nasal vowels are located they can be used as target models for improved resonance even though the pitch temporarily may not be appropriate. From these non-nasal target sounds work can proceed towards normal resonance in the optimum pitch range.

Where rate is concerned, slowing down or speeding up may be required. Greene (1980) suggested that people with hypernasality should use slowed speech. Alternatively, other workers reported a study which showed that normal speakers are perceived as more nasal when speaking slower than their normal rate.

Vocal abuse may also be detected in speakers with hypernasality, especially those attempting to increase modal loudness levels.

This problem should be dealt with as previously described always taking into account the need to eliminate the presence of an organic factor, by referring to the ENT specialist.

Facial grimaces and nostril flaring may be present in some cases of hypernasality. These habits may arise from repeated attempts to prevent or minimize nasal emission of sound. Mirror work, negative practice and teaching light, quick articulation contacts will all help to eliminate, or at least reduce, grimacing and flaring.

Van Riper (1973) stated that velopharyngeal muscles can be strengthened by the use of physical exercises if any degree of closure is possible.

Reduction of tension can be achieved by relaxation such as that suggested by Moncur and Brackett (1974):

1. relax mandible and tongue;
2. aim for maximum downward movement of mandible and tongue for vowel production;
3. concentrate on keeping the pharyngo-oral tract relaxed and open;
4. ensure good breath support;
5. pause between syllables for unhurried inhalation, e.g. 'rah, rah, rah' *pause* 'yaw yaw yaw' *pause* 'ahm ahm ahm' *pause* 'ohm ohm ohm'.

It has been noted by several workers that tension increases with fatigue and this should be considered in all circumstances.

The correction of breath direction can be facilitated by using musical instruments; holding air under pressure in the mouth by blowing out the cheeks, holding the nostrils if necessary, and alternating oral and nasal emission of air (p. 28), consciously opening the mouth wider to permit a higher proportion of oral resonance to nasal resonance. Practise deliberate yawning, intoning, singing, blowing using different oral postures, e.g. place upper teeth on lower lip, blow air interrupting it with /f/ and /v/. It is useful to use negative practice with the latter exercises.

Improved resonance will follow attention to activity of mouth, tongue and mandible. Tongue and lip exercises should begin with oral gymnastics, e.g. starting with sensory awareness as previously described, and progressing to clean-cut motor movement. Sometimes it is useful to introduce a palatal lift or a palatal stimulator to decrease the velopharyngeal gap. The purpose is to stimulate movement away from the device. To exercise the soft palate the use of /ŋ/ is recommended. Using some of their procedures Stemple (1984) devised the following sequence with mirror work:

1. Pant vigorously while watching rise and fall of the soft palate in a mirror, then practise raising the soft palate without panting and vocalizing.
2. Yawn slowly observing movement of soft palate – repeat without yawning.
3. Raise palate and say /ɑ/ prolonging the vowel, keeping the palate raised say words beginning with /ɑ/ such as 'are', 'army'.
4. Say word with final /ŋ/ such as 'bang', prolonging the /ŋ/ and noting how the back of the tongue humps up against the palate. Now say /ŋ/ and blend it into /ɑ/ keeping the soft palate raised.

Swallowing exercises

There is disagreement about the effectiveness of swallowing exercises to improve velopharyngeal closure and therefore reduce hypernasality. Studies have supported both arguments. Experience shows that individual differences again influence the outcome of such exercises. Some clients benefit, others do not. These exercises usually include blowing exercises with or without using a manometer or other similar blowing device, demonstrate sucking through a straw or with a meter to indicate pressure and finally swallowing practice. Monitoring swallowing movements by placing the index finger on the neck in the area of the thyroid cartilage can be demonstrated. Swallowing time may be increased by stopping momentarily just after beginning to swallow and then continuing swallowing. In some clients this method leads to better velopharyngeal closure.

Regular and frequent swallowing practice can prove an appropriate part of a programme devised to improve functional hypernasality and resonance imbalance in clients with submucous cleft or palatal paralysis.

HYPONASALITY

This condition frequently arises following surgical intervention for the removal of nasal obstructions such as adenoids or nasal polyps.

Surgery to remove the offending obstruction is rarely sufficient to reduce the hyponasality, as the habit factor has usually been firmly established. Specific resonance balance has to be achieved as recommended for hypernasality (p. 124). On this occasion the therapist uses a hyponasal voice. The next step is to instruct the client how and when to use nasal sounds. Production of /m/, /n/ and /ŋ/ follows. These sounds should then be practised in words, phrases, sentences and connected speech. The use of nasal blowing (p. 127), and placing the fingers on both sides of the bridge of the nose to feel the vibrations transmitted from the nasal cavity, are recommended as aids to learning. Increasing the phonation time on these sounds in connected speech decreases the impression of hyponasality. Listening training is a vital component of treatment as the user must be able to correct by self-monitoring.

In cases of chronically open eustachian tubes, auditory feedback is altered resulting in hyponasality and autophony. The latter phenomenon is due to the speaker's voice reaching both sides of the eardrum simultaneously so that he/she perceives his voice as having hollow rainbarrel resonance. Occasionally occluding the external auditory canals provides temporary relief from autophony. Another technique is to have a person monitor his/her amplified voice through earphones to provide a cancelling effect on sounds reaching the middle ear from both sides of the eardrum. The client must be highly motivated to learn to tolerate and accept autophony and benefit from clinical intervention.

Elimination of facial grimaces and nares (nostril) construction in hyponasality as in hypernasality provides cosmetic improvement. Modifying and eliminating vocal abuse and establishing balanced muscular tonus are necessary for improving the quality of the laryngeal tone. Adequate speech intelligibility should be the prime objective from the listener's viewpoint and optimum balanced resonance that of the speaker.

CLOSED HEAD INJURY

Dysphonias of varying severity may result from closed head injury. Post-traumatic mutism may be followed by severe breathiness, which often persists after articulatory recovery. Sapir and Aronson (1985) describe two such patients and postulate that their dysphonia may have been due to a frontal lobe-limbic system disturbance, which affected their motivation, personality and judgement. Such neural disturbances are said to be responsible, among other things, for apathy, lack of drive, 'flat' vocal-facial expressions of emotion and affect, and poor insight into the inappropriateness of vocal and non-vocal behaviours. In the first patient, good speech, language and cognitive skills were reported after therapy, although the patient retained mild memory deficits, mild residual left hemiparesis and nearly complete left homonymous hemianopia. Treatment for the dysphonia in this case was the use of symptomatic voice therapy used for conversion therapy (Aronson, 1985):

1. Pressure was exerted bilaterally to the thyroid cartilage, working the larynx downward while the client coughed on command. Her voice when she coughed was described as 'nice and loud'.
2. Pressure was again applied while the client cleared her throat. 'Good phonation' was commented on once more.
3. Next, the client was asked to clear her throat and say /ɑ/, still with digital pressure. This was repeated several times until near normal phonation was achieved.
4. Counting from 1–20 was started and digital pressure added intermittently during the count.
5. Conversational practice supported at first with pressure and later with spoken encouragement followed, until eventually a reasonably breathy-free voice was established.

The second case, a man of 22 years of age, suffered a severe closed head injury which necessitated surgery and from which the patient made a very slow recovery. More than a month after injury he began to show signs of comprehending speech and eventually to respond with a few whispered words. Once again symptomatic voice therapy was used and produced consistent phonation very quickly. Prosody and facial expression were 'flat'. Vocal volume was achieved within a few days but prosody remained 'flat'. Both patients with post-traumatic dysphonia regained their voices within one session of symptomatic voice therapy. Sapir and Aronson (1985) repeated that specific neural damage was difficult to determine in those two particular cases.

ROAD TRAFFIC ACCIDENT

Acquired dysphonia may be a result of a Road Traffic Accident (RTA). It may be caused by oedema, in which case a reasonable prognosis can be made, as eventually, with the reduction of inflammation and swelling, the vocal folds will return to normal or near-normal. Alternatively, dysphonia may be characteristic of nerve damage at upper or lower motor neurone levels. Recovery will then depend on the severity and permanence of the damage. Scholefield (1987), has described three cases of aphonia following closed head injury. One had vocal fold oedema, and different types of nerve damage appeared to cause the others. The tentative conclusion drawn from this study postulated that the dysphonia involved both the limbic system and the right hemisphere, and that emotional phonation and emotional facial expression were absent. This investigation particularly supports the case for specific management to meet the needs of the various possible deficits in voice, speech and language which can result from an RTA. Similar disorders may arise from other traumas and require similar treatment methods.

LARYNGECTOMY

Management of laryngectomy is one of the most difficult for the speech therapist, as the responsibility of facilitating an alternative means of phonation is the focus of treatment. Surgery to remove larynxes usually damaged by cancerous growths has been successfully recorded since 1874. Where the neoplasm is contained within the larynx total physical recovery is possible. Pharyngolaryngectomy and, in severe cases, oesophagopharyngolaryngectomy may be required depending on the penetration of the cancerous growth. In each case, however, the patient is left without the means to phonate. Attempts to provide air for fluent speech have been sought by several means. The difficulty has always been the dual function of shunt, to facilitate an uninterrupted airflow while being resistant to aspiration of food and liquids.

In 1980, Singer and Blom introduced their successful one-stage procedure with a single one-way valved voice prosthesis. This innovation has solved many earlier problems. Over time this tracheo-oesophageal (TE) 'puncture' technique has been modified. As with oesophageal voice, TE 'puncture' voice relies on a

131

tonic pharyngeal-oesophageal (PE) segment to act as vibrator for voice production. Videofluoroscopy has provided a great deal of information regarding the function of the PE segment. As a result it is now possible to categorize laryngectomees into five different groups: hypotonic, tonic, hypertonic, spasm and stricture.

A study carried out at a monthly Laryngectomy Voice Clinic at Charing Cross Hospital, London, during 1983–87 is described by Perry (1988). There were 166 subjects of whom 36, the 'primary' series, underwent laryngectomy during which a surgically created tracheo-oesophageal fistula was made. Ten days later a prosthesis was fitted. The remaining 130 participants, the 'secondary' series, had undergone surgery months, and in some cases years, previously and were interested in improving their communication by having the Singer-Blom procedure carried out. After counselling, 81 clients remained in the 'secondary' series. Management was carried out in ways appropriate to the needs of both groups of patients.

Those subjects in the 'primary' series were given liquids 9 or 10 days after surgery. If no aspiration of fluid occurred through the neck repair, semisolid food was introduced the next day. The Ryle's tube was removed if no breakdown of the surgical repair occurred after a day of eating. The speech therapist then sized and fitted a Singer-Blom silicone prosthesis of the requisite length. Two weeks after the initial surgery and three days after the prosthesis was fitted each laryngectomee was able to maintain and manage it, and was transferred to outpatient care. Three months later 34 of the 36 patients were still using their prostheses as their sole means of communication. The two failed speakers were both foreign and used their prosthesis well initially. However, within 3 months of returning to their own countries the prostheses were extruded, having been inadvertently pulled out while clearing mucus, and they were unable to replace them soon enough to avoid the fistula closing. This can occur within 10 minutes of removal.

Of the 16 hypotonic patients in the 'secondary' series, 12 elected to have a TE puncture and seven of these were successful. Alcoholism (one case), poor visual acuity (two cases) and disliking the speech quality (two cases) accounted for the failure of the other 5 cases. In the tonic group, 11 of the 18 subjects opted for a TE puncture and nine were successful. Again, two cases disliked the speech quality, feeling that it was not an improvement over their previous ability. Both had irregularly shaped neck contours which may have accounted for their inability to wear an external tracheostomy valve for hands-free voicing. Of the 34 patients in the hypertonic group, 24 opted for the TE puncture but none agreed to the extra myotomy which was deemed necessary for this group. Consequently, 19 succeeded with the use of a low pressure prosthesis. Of the five who were unsuccessful, two developed complications, one was alcoholic, one prosthesis extruded and was not replaced quickly enough and one disliked the speech quality.

In the group with spasm, 27 of the 54 underwent a myotomy and a TE puncture and two opted for a puncture alone. Success occurred with 24 subjects. Of the five failures, two disliked the voice quality, one extruded and was not replaced quickly enough and in the two who did not have the myotomy performed, the prostheses used were of too high a resistance to allow air to flow into the pharynx. (The failure of these two subjects led to the development of the videofluoroscopic classification and, since its implementation, the success rate has risen significantly.) In the group of eight subjects with stricture, three had additional surgery as well as the TE puncture and two had the TE puncture alone.

Results showed much higher successes in the 'primary' series, 94%, compared with 79% in the 'secondary' series. However, the latter is considerably higher than reports of successful oesophageal speech previously recorded. Part of the success is due to careful categorization of the subjects which ensures that they receive maximum differential treatment according to their needs (Perry and Edels, 1985). Oesophageal speech is still a possible achievement after TE intervention. Factors which influence the outcome of treatment with laryngectomees include age, general health, physical state of the oral, pharyngeal and oesophageal tissue, attitude to the situation, motivation to produce an acceptable voice and family and other support.

At a recent seminar, one of the five or six given in different parts of the country each year, sponsored by Cancer Relief and organized by the National Association of Laryngectomee Clubs, emphasis was placed on contemporary surgical procedures and techniques. Although most of the discussion referred to the Singer-Blom punctures, mention was made of other similar approaches. Primary versus secondary punctures were debated and the importance of assessment stressed. Rehabilitation programmes rely heavily on aiming for good quality of life. This has been made easier by the involvement in every area of patients willing to interchange experiences and facilitate the greatest possible improvement in each other's communicative progress.

AGEING

Management of speech difficulties in the ageing again falls into the categories already referred to: normal, continuation of developmental disorders and acquired disorders.

Normal

Knowledge of the biological changes in ageing is a prerequisite for the understanding of all other aspects of change taking place (Bromley, 1974). Much of the brain is concerned with one or other aspect of communication, language, speech, gestural and body language. It appears that age-related neuronal loss takes place, according to some experts. This would account for limits being placed on the continuing ability to maintain 'spot-on' communicative ability. Not only does this appear to affect memory but also motor skills. Ramig (1986) describes the speech used by the elderly as being:

slow, with long pauses and hesitancy
reduced in intelligibility
having increased silent time
having increased duration of phonemes.

As in all other age groups, the elderly include well-maintained individuals and those who are less well-maintained. Chronologically 'old' people may continue to be physiologically 'young'. However, in the normal speech dyad the concept of 'old' speech is more in the ear of the listener than in the mouth of the speaker.

It is just as important to carry out careful assessment at this stage as at any other stage in life. Sometimes assessment reveals the adoption of poor physical habits. Counselling may be the main managerial approach, where this occurs. Attitudes to older people will have to improve if the country is to operate successfully in a future in which a considerable proportion of the population is approaching, or over, 'official' retirement age.

In a world of 'isms', ageism is pervasive throughout society. Greene *et al.* (1986), describing doctor/elderly patient relations in the USA, stated that specific assumptions about older people are legion, e.g. they can't hear, they can't remember, they can't think for themselves, they are depressing, they are non-productive, they are infantile. Greene *et al.* describe a study conducted by two social scientists and two doctors in a major urban teaching hospital in New York. Five physicians were audio-taped, each interviewing eight patients, four young and four elderly. Each doctor's group was matched for race and sex. Ten more doctors were taped interviewing an additional four elderly patients each. This extra data was collected to allow further study of doctor/elderly patient encounters. Topics were limited to four categories: medical, personal habits, psycho-social and other.

Results showed that differences in response areas were largely attributable to *physician behaviour*. Several hypotheses reflecting anecdotal assumptions of the medical literature were disproved by the data. Non-specific problems of living were *not* mentioned more often by elderly patients than by younger. Medical issues were found to predominate in the discussions with both groups. Particular areas of interest like dentures, constipation and hearingloss were *not* introduced more often by the elderly group as was predicted. No signs of the repetitious, boring older patient were apparent. Elderly patients did prove less able than younger ones to get their specific points over. This suggested a diminution of assertiveness to the researchers who suggested that it should be followed up to determine whether this is an area in which older people should be given help. Elderly people also appeared to 'play according to the rules' more than younger ones do. Other interesting points were made in this vein. Further research of this type is required to clarify the points to be dealt with to improve the situation.

Personal experience with an ailing parent in a doctor/patient relationship illustrated the 'does he take sugar' effect, in which the patient was not addressed directly, but through his daughter. The patient was completely *compos mentis* until he died three years later. Such examples indicate that the focus of management must be placed on the social attitudes of the younger to the older members of the population.

Education should include allusions to the physical frailty of ageing the the presence of clarity of mind and vast life experience. Too many old people appear to die in a state of depression having become convinced that they are unloved and unwanted. Many suffer years of fear and worry for their safety from young vandals and muggers. Others experience unbearable loneliness, possibly in physical comfort but in emotional isolation from family and friends. This state of affairs has become established and should be faced and reconsidered. Often the first indication that someone has fallen into this category is the loss of motor speed and efficiency after many years of physical independence. Professionals, such as physiotherapists, occupational therapists, speech therapists, psychologists and social workers, are so over-burdened with caring for the more active members of society that they unwittingly, and often unwillingly, fail to provide adequate cover for this section of the community. Provision of centres where all aspects of living are catered for are available abroad. For example, in Canada centres exist where 'honoured citizens', as they are sometimes called, can join in and help to run all kinds of physical and recreational activities in buildings where medical, social, cosmetic and other types of helpful services are available under one roof. Independence is the operative aim. The continued use of skills is often the best maintenance of them. Age does not negate the importance of competitiveness, purpose and inter-change of ideas and experiences. These considerations are not directly relevant to speech production but they are appropriate to all ageing individuals and each aspect of development has to be viewed in the general context of everyday life.

The most common physical weaknesses in speech of the later years affect articulation and phonation. Slowed movements demand more deliberate use of muscles and, where intelligibility becomes involved, exercises similar to those used in dysarthria and dysphonia may be beneficial. It is seldom necessary to practise such exercises in normal deterioration. The overall slowing-down process which occurs enables most older speakers to adjust their speech production to their capabilities.

Continuation of developmental disorders

Disablement of all kinds in the past led to shorter life expectancy. Nowadays, with the advance of medical and social welfare, many individuals in this category can expect to live into old age. Research into older people with Down's syndrome (DS) indicates that many survive into their fifth decade and some are still living beyond 60. Studies reveal a tendency for them to develop Alzheimer's disease at an earlier age and more frequently *pro rata* than the normal population. Sylvester (1983) found neuropathological features similar to those of Alzheimer's disease, in 88.9% of patients with DS over 30 years of age, 95% over 40 years and 100% over 50 years. The implications of these findings for the production of speech are mostly concerned with increased dysarthric symptoms which, in turn, affect levels of intelligibility. Management problems in this situation may also be present, due to the linguistic and intellectual deterioration which also result from Alzheimer's. Therapeutic intervention may be difficult for these clients due to the reduction in comprehension of, and memory for, the instructions necessary to explain therapy techniques.

Normalization, as described previously, may produce problems for older people with mental handicap, as the ageing process has not been fully studied in this area and, it seems, would inevitably lead to greater difficulties than those experienced by normally ageing people. When individuals become unintelligible, or fail to replace their poorer articulatory abilities with other forms of communication, their independence becomes further threatened. Provision may have to be made for such individuals. People with mental handicap usually require back-up sessions of treatment throughout their lives to maintain the progress they have made. With ageing, this will become even more necessary and efforts to supply clinicians and resources will have to be increased.

Groups of older people with mental handicap can be encouraged to partake in sessions of music and movement to build up and maintain good breathing habits, relaxed movements and to improve their general physical state. In the course of exercising, implicit speech treatment can be included by using spoken, sung and chanted accompaniments, a continuation of the 'directive function of speech' (Luria, 1973), or 'rhythmic intention' (Harri and Tillemans, 1984). Concurrently, with the most severely handicapped people, continued use of appropriate materials such as those constructed by Caldwell (pp. 113–4) is indicated (personal communication).

For people with physical handicaps, the prevention of deformities should always be a priority. The management team of physical, occupational and speech therapists, working in their specialist areas, should make a planned, concerted approach to maintain near-normal function.

One specific aspect which should be considered by the speech therapist is oral hygiene and dental requirements. Frequently, good speech production is expected from an individual who could attain a much better performance if the hygenic state of her/his mouth and dentition have been examined and improved (Appendix C). If the dental needs involve dentures, the availability of the prosthesis does not mean that improvement will follow. It is almost always necessary to make several adjustments to achieve a good 'fit'. Many people elect to take the easy way out and do not persevere with the dentures after they have been supplied. Not only does this lead to alterations in facial structure, but also it 'dampens down' articulation and detracts from chewing. If, at a much earlier stage, little or no attempt has been made to encourage the person who is disabled to take a pride in her/his appearance, it will not be easy to insist on them making an effort at this point, but it should be tried. In the physically disabled it is important to maintain good breathing patterns, and, of course, good posture. Health, strength and the ability to produce clear speech will benefit. A programme based on ideal physical conditions, or at least the optimum for each individual (which should have been established in earlier life), will not produce maximum results, but nevertheless should be implemented.

Augmentative or compensatory systems introduced and established earlier should be checked and modified. People who have been using Makaton, for instance, may be able to derive more benefit from the addition of Makaton symbols to widen their communicative ability. In cases where deformities have developed, alternative means may have to be tried.

Where the muscles have become weaker with advancing age, a synthesizer or other suitable communication aid may be found to boost attempts at communication. Intensive assessment is available at Communication Aid Centres to enable engineers, therapists and other specialists to plan, construct and apply modified aids to enable disabled people to maximize what little normal function they may have. Technology has facilitated this service and has, for example, been used to fit an appliance to an ankle, wrist or head which can activate some form of signal to drive a sophisticated communication aid. A degree of independence may be achieved by such methods by enabling the individual to ring a bell, open a door, switch on TV, stereo, radio, tea-maker or whatever form of equipment may be required. Work is going ahead on the use of speech to activate such appliances. The clinician can be instrumental in helping to provide the individual with the necessary speech production for this purpose.

Acquired disorders

Disease and trauma occur most often in ageing individuals. The diseases which affect the production of speech are either infections and breakdowns in the vocal tract, or those resulting from neuronal changes in the brain. The former include lung-related disorders such as *emphysema*, which can take the form of an alveolar distension in the pulmonary tissues, and which interferes with breathing and so affects voice and speech production, *bronchitis* has the same effect on voice and speech. *Neoplasms* may occur within the lungs, bronchi, trachea, larynx, pharynx, oral and nasal cavities and any of the organs within these cavities such as the tongue. Cranial nerve defect(s) may arise, for example:

1. the trigeminal (V) affecting the face, nose and mouth;
2. the facial (VII) affecting the muscles of expression;
3. the glossopharyngeal (XI) affecting the muscles of the tongue and the throat;
4. the vagus (X) affecting the pharyngeal and laryngeal muscles;
5. the hypoglossal (XII) affecting the muscles of the tongue.

Damage, as the result of infection or assault to any of these nerves will affect the production of speech to a lesser or greater degree. Frequently there is recovery from this type of nerve damage and normal use of muscles becomes possible once more.

As mentioned previously, thyroid imbalance may occur and disrupt the production of speech. This can occur at any period of life. Management of all these conditions is similar to that already described and dependent on the total physical condition of each individual.

The more common types of illness found in older people derive from cerebral damage or dysfunction. Examples of the latter are *Parkinson's disease*, *lower motor neurone disease*, *myasthenia gravis*, all of which affect the muscular systems of the body. Research has led to some amelioration in Parkinson's syndrome by medication. This can decrease the tremor, particularly of the hands and, to some degree, of the tongue, which compounds the overall muscle weakness which so badly affects articulation. Prosodic features are disrupted and the personal aspects of reduced speech affecting intelligibility. Here again, selective exercises have to be tried to find the most effective means of implementing improvement. Current research has led to experimental transplant surgery in which relevant fetal brain tissue is implanted in the Parkinson's patient's brain in the hope of regrowth of normal tissue. It is too early to judge the degree of success for this method. The issue in this type of surgery raises many moral and ethical points which may never be fully resolved.

Some of these conditions do not respond to any known treatment and in *lower motor neurone disease*, for example, the whole muscular system eventually stops functioning. Where actual damage is inflicted as the result of a *cerebral vascular accident (CVA)* such as *thrombosis, haemorrhage, aneurysm* or *embolism* in the left hemisphere of the brain, language can be disrupted to some extent. Usually this damage leads to some breakdown in both the comprehension and expression of language, that is, the individual has difficulty in decoding heard language and in formulating appropriate responses to heard language, or in initiating language for him/herself (dysphasia).

In the latter case, where expressive language is affected, there is quite often an associated disruption in the articulation of speech – acquired dyspraxia. When present to a severe degree this can be a most debilitating disorder. When this persists beyond the point of spontaneous recovery, there is no known treatment for the condition and an alternative system of communication may have to be taught. In very old patients, this can prove too difficult and little communicative progress may be possible. This state of affairs leads to problems in hospital and the home and may result in a most depressed patient and family.

The patient may, however, have access to written or computed language in some instances. Management should include as many sessions of treatment as possible in the early stages, twice per day is ideal, in an attempt to recover as much ground as possible, during the period of spontaneous recovery.

Experience has shown that the damage caused by a CVA can be compared to a severe cut on the surface of the skin surrounded by an area of bruising. The scar which will eventually be left by the cut represents the group of neurones which will not recover, but the bruised area will disappear. Therapy facilitates the best possible means of ridding the client of the bruising and at the same time learning strategies to compensate for the scar. CVA can be preceded and followed by transient ischaemic episodes – small, short-lived, stroke-like attacks – during which speech may be lost or disrupted for short periods of time. Mostly, total ability returns but occasionally some aspects of language and/or speech may be lost. It is always useful to have an assessment made of returned function to determine whether future management may be indicated following any further episode(s). *Pseudobulbar palsy* results from bilateral CVAs and resultant dysarthria is frequently dense in nature. Feeding, particularly swallowing, is often specifically affected and tube feeding may have to be adopted until restored power returns to the muscles. The muscles of articulation may be less severely affected in such patients and speech may be reasonably intelligible.

Possibly the greatest disruption of communication in the elderly results from *Alzheimer's disease* (p. 108). Speech, as opposed to language, is less often affected and just as the patient continues to use normal motor skills for walking, sitting, eating she/he can produce clearly enunciated speech patterns. The communication difficulty is confined to semantic and pragmatic aspects of language, that is, appropriate meaningfulness and the use of language is affected.

In addition to severe illnesses and disorders, older people may develop several minor ailments which react to early treatment. The tendency in some doctors to ignore such conditions, or equate them with normal ageing and do nothing about them, has to be guarded against. Good medical care can extend comfort and ease difficulties at this period of life as at every other.

Intelligible automatic forms of language may be produced by patients in a comatose state after a considerable period. This illustrates the continuing efficiency of the automatic sensory feedback loop systems which activate the movements of the muscle groups necessary for the *production of speech*. Many people in history are remembered best for their 'last words'. Thus, right up to the point of death human beings can maintain their uniqueness by being able to exert some influence by means of speech.

141

Appendix A

BASIC EXERCISES (BE)

1. Discuss with the parent/carer/teacher the need for oral, nasal and dental hygiene.

    (a) With a cotton bud dipped in diluted antiseptic (e.g. TCP or Dettol) clean the tongue surfaces and lateral areas between the tongue and the cheeks.

    (b) Clean the teeth with toothpaste on a toothbrush using vertical movements and simultaneously massaging the gums.

    (c) Start nose-blowing exercises; with a tissue between your thumb and index finger gently grasp the child's nose. Close off one nostril with pressure from your thumb and ask the child to blow down the other nostril while moving your index finger backward and forward against the side of the open nostril. Repeat with the other nostril.

    After habitual mouth breathing this may be difficult for the child and careful instruction to the parent plus some form of reward system may be necessary. However, the improvement that comes with success makes perseverance worthwhile. Be prepared to provide a great deal of support to both the parent and the child.

    The aim is for the child to carry out the whole action for her/himself.

2. Instruct the parent in and demonstrate central breathing using full inter-costal diaphragmatic movements. Repeat over several visits until the parent has felt the benefit and is motivated to pass the technique on to the child.

3. Encourage the parent to demonstrate and practise central breathing with the child.
4. To promote flexibility of the lower costal muscles, practise:
   (a) Breathing in swinging the arms backward, forward, backward; breathing out, swinging arms forward and straight up above the head calling out loudly 'out' to expel all the breath. Repeat the movements in rhythmic succession, i.e. immediately 'out' has been called, swing the arms downward and backward again.
   (b) Breathing in, raising the arms outward and sideways to shoulder level; breathing out, swinging the arms down and up to the opposite shoulders, so that they cross in front of the body; as they cross expel all the breath by loudly shouting 'out'. Repeat the movements with a smooth swinging rhythm, i.e. as soon as 'out' has been called, swing the arms down and up to shoulder level again.
5. Proceed by showing the parent how to increase breath control.
   (a) Fill the lungs with breath in a relaxed fashion.
   (b) Hold the breath in the lungs momentarily.
   (c) Exhale the breath on a softly articulated /f/ or /s/.
   (d) Repeat (a) and (b) then exhale the breath counting to 1–2–3–4–5 using an intoned chant.
   (e) Increase controlled exhalation by counting to 10, 15, 20 and so on until maximum level is reached.
6. Encourage the parent to demonstrate this technique to the child.

Appendix B

SPACE, TIME AND SEQUENCING

1. Check that the child is aware of the limits of his/her body in space as follows:
   (a) stand still and lift both arms above the head;
   (b) stand still and lift both arms out to the sides;
   (c) stand still, then bend down to touch the floor;
   (d) roll on the floor, feeling and identifying all the perimeters of the body;
   (e) sit with the child, side by side in front of a mirror.
      (i) each point to your hair, nose, eyes, mouth
      (ii) each point to your arms, legs, back, stomach
      (iii) each point to your left elbow, right knee
      (iv) identify your wrists, ankles, eyebrows, and so on
      (v) identify each other's facial and body parts by pointing
      (vi) proceed to naming the body parts including less obvious ones, e.g. the lobe of your left ear.
2. Check comprehension of spatial language: up, down, under, over, in, on, above, beside, between, near, far, in front of, in the middle, behind, on top, underneath, inside, outside, here, there, where. Learn by active use. Do not ask the child to say words.
3. Copy patterns. Count steps between objects. Identify figure/-foreground/background. Incorporate appropriate sections of the Frostig Programme on Spatial Relationships (Frostig and Horne, 1966). (See Teachers' Guide, pp. 161–4.)
4. Practise tasks of visuo-motor sequencing, e.g.
   (a) copying sequences of beads, blocks, dominoes
   (b) reproducing written letters, numbers colours
   (c) solving mazes

(d) copying patterns and pictures by joining the appropriate dots.

5. Check the child's awareness of temporal attributes: now, then, before, after, as soon as, immediately, later, today, tomorrow, yesterday, days, weeks, months, years, seasons as appropriate. The tenses of verbs may have to be learned consciously.

6. Sequencing. Adopt a strict daily routine including organized preparation for:
   (a) washing: ensure that materials are always available
   (b) dressing: help the child to lay out her/his clothes in order of putting on
   (c) breakfast: at the table with all provisions available
   (d) brushing teeth: aim for the child to make this a proficient, automatic habit
   (e) play/TV
       helping Mum   } for the pre-school child
       walks/shopping
       leaving for school   for the schoolchild.

7. Cooperate with friends, relatives, playgroup/nursery school leaders and teachers. Discuss with all involved the best means of sequencing all familiar tasks.

8. Plan home activities, including areas of responsibility, e.g. stacking, washing and drying dishes; selecting and laying out clothes for the morning.

9. Use familiar repetitive language to name common objects, e.g. body schema; comics/storybooks/pictures.

10. Vocalize by humming; singing; repeating nursery rhymes; reading stories.

11. Recognize learning modalities (sight, hearing, feeling, touch) and modify the strategies that the child uses.

12. Stimulate listening and watching in everyday contexts. Check that the child comprehends instructions, functions and purposes of everyday objects. Encourage the child to question and understand new experiences and the stages required to learn them and thus increase skills.

13. Utilize strategies by which the child can learn and remember techniques to make sequencing easier, e.g. mark the inside of shoes with coloured Xs to enable the child to put them together in order to put them on the correct feet.

14. Sort picture sequences of everyday activities, increasing the complexity as task becomes easier.

15. Enable the child to sort out spatial and other relationships.

16. Proceed to language sequencing where necessary.

145

Appendix C

ORAL MECHANISM EXAMINATION

1. Seat the child comfortably in an upright position in a chair which enables the clinician to be on eye-level with the child's mouth. The head should be held in the natural mid-line with the chin pulled slightly in and down.
2. Check that the head is of normal size and that the face is symmetrical. Note any anomalous characteristics. In a normally developing face there should be balance between the two sides, eyes should be at the same level, of normally acceptable size, neither too closely nor too distantly set; the nose should be roughly in the mid-line with a straight septal division; the mouth should be closed at rest and gentle, regular nasal breathing should be present; the face should be divided approximately into three:
   (a) between the hairline and the bridge of the nose;
   (b) between the bridge of the nose and the upper lip;
   (c) between the upper lip and the point of the chin.
   Normal occlusion of the jaws should allow for the absence of upper or lower thrust. Specific characteristics such as epicanthic folds of the eyelids, Brushfield spots in the iris, squint(s), nystagmus or other peculiarities of the eyes or other facial features should be noted.
3. Observe the child's use of the speech mechanism. Organs may appear to function adequately in isolation but fail to interact and relate in dynamic performance. Many children with speech and language disorders adopt habits such as posturing of their lips and/or tongue. Check as follows:

146

Lips

(a) Are they always apart?
(b) Is closure possible? (This depends on whether the sensori-motor function is normal and whether the nose is clear to permit normal nasal breathing.) (Appendix A.)
(c) Has the child adopted a smiling posture of the lips? (This may be due to the child having learned that when one has difficulty in making people understand it is more acceptable to look pleasant by wearing a perpetual smile. The effect of this is to distort further the productions of segments which are already abnormal and so increase unintelligibility. Considerable time may be spent in reversing this habit. Attitude change is usually the answer as the cause is psychological rather than physical. This is an example of the importance of 'talking out' the whole problem with the child.)
(d) Is there continual protrusion or retraction of the lips?
(e) Is there frequent licking of the lips?
(f) Severe lip scarring after cleft-lip surgery may have surprisingly little effect on articulation. Children expedite numerous means of compensating for physical disabilities. Experience shows that inability to use the lips competently depends more on getting other aspects right, such as breathing. Test lips by asking child to protrude, retract, open and close them.

Tongue

This may be an unruly member in a quite different context from the biblical one. Anomalies of the tongue include:

(a) Tongue thrust: this traditionally has been seen as the result of incomplete establishment of adult swallow patterns, that is, persistence of the infantile forward projection of the tongue required for sucking. In many instances this positioning of the tongue beyond the expected age has very little effect on the production of articulation. Occasionally, however, this feature in combination with other immature patterns, interferes with the clear production of articulation and thence with the completely normal development of a phonological system.

It also hinders the development of adult feeding patterns. Warner (1981) advises specific means of holding the spoon for children with feeding problems resulting from tongue thrust. ('For a tongue thrust put the bowl of the spoon on the front of the tongue and press down gently and at the same time slightly back' (p. 43).)

Observation of the child eating and drinking is essential for the clinician to determine the extensiveness of the thrust.

Dentition may be adversely affected due to the continual pressure of the tongue on the growing teeth. Certain factors will influence both the timing and the usefulness of treatment for tongue thrust. Children with one or more of the following habits will be less likely to benefit from treatment:

  (i) consistent mouth breathing
 (ii) thumb or finger sucking
(iii) a high or narrow arched palate
 (iv) various open-, cross- or over-bites
  (v) enlarged tonsils, adenoids and other nasal obstructions.

Orthodontic intervention, desensitization of nasal allergies, removal of chronically inflamed and enlarged tonsils and adenoids are some means by which nasal breathing, lip closure and readiness for treatment for tongue thrust can be achieved. In the US, infrequent surgical intervention to reduce tongue size is performed. Experience shows that such intervention is counter-productive. Speech therapy often produces the necessary improvements, by encouraging more normal tongue positioning.

(b) Fissures: these do not usually interfere with speech but may upset resonance.
(c) Tongue-tie: this is rarely severe enough to be treated but may require conscious production of certain combinations of tongue movement, e.g. those in words such as 'preliminary'.
(d) Macroglossia: this is usually due to oedema, neoplasm or allergic reactions.
(e) Microglossia: a rare condition in which the tongue is remarkably small but usually still able to produce accept-

able articulation. Test tongue as follows: elevate, depress, move laterally, move in a circular motion over the surface of the lips.

Jaws

Most problems are of an orthodontic nature, i.e. caused by an inferior or superior misalignment:
(a) malocclusion due to overshooting of maxilla;
(b) malocclusion due to undershooting of the mandible, in both cases jaw movement may be limited and referral to an orthodontist should be made;
(c) some children are unable to carry out lateral movements of the jaw, e.g. in dyspraxia, when the difficulty results from inability to initiate the movement voluntarily.
Test jaw as follows: observe alignment, closure; move laterally and vertically.

Palate

(a) This may be cleft, either complete, partial or in the form of a sub-mucous cleft.
(b) The velum may be unnaturally short and fail to meet the pharyngeal wall.
(c) A degree of paralysis or weakness may be present due to a neurological lesion
Such conditions will result in a disorder of resonance.
Test palate as follows: observe and feel surface; listen to quality of resonance, produce /ŋ/ and /ŋa/ repeatedly.

Nose

(a) Observe septum for mid-line straightness.
(b) Note condition of nasal bridge, particularly observing a 'spreading, flattened tendency'.
(c) Where apparent blockage is present ascertain that the nostrils can be clear on occasion. If this is never the case, refer to the GP for examination for possible choanal atresia (lack

of posterior openings leading to cul-de-sac resonance). Nasal polyps or other neoplasms may be present.

Vocal Folds

(a) Listen for breathiness, hoarseness, and pitch.
(b) Observe breathing and method used.
(c) Note general body posture and, in particular, head, neck and shoulder posture.
(d) Assess tongue and jaw position.
(e) Check vocal attack, vocal support, voice onset time.
(f) Listen for voice placement, projection and quality.
(g) Use electrolaryngography, electromyography and/or X-rays where appropriate.

Appendix D

FEEDING/EATING TECHNIQUES

1. Position the client in the best seated position with his/her head in the midline, and held slightly forward (controlled if necessary).
2. Check that the mouth is clean:
   (a) with wet finger, starting at the midline run the finger to corner of the mouth and enter the mouth;
   (b) feel around inside one cheek noting the muscle tone, smoothness of surface, presence of food;
   (c) repeat on the other side of the mouth.
3. Stroke the face on both sides from the cheeks to the corners of the mouth to reduce hypersensitivity. To achieve this within the mouth, hold the jaw open and, gently, but firmly, rub the gums, alveolar ridge and the palate. Where a strong bite reflex is present, do this with the back of a polythene spoon.
4. Present small quantities of food, using a polythene spoon, at the midline of the mouth. Avoid scraping the upper tooth and stimulating the bite reflex when removing the spoon.
5. Close the lips and jaw and place two fingers, one above the upper and one below the lower lip, to maintain a seal.
6. Move the jaw in a circular motion to stimulate chewing.
7. Encourage swallowing by stroking a finger along the underside of the chin towards the neck. This movement raises the back of the tongue.
8. If necessary, have client turn or tilt head until tongue has the bolus under control.
9. Only present more food when the mouth is empty. Give small

drinks of iced water during the meal to refresh the mouth and stimulate swallowing.

10. To improve drinking, liquid should be given in a cup with the rim placed between the lips, while the jaw is supported to prevent excessive movement.

11. Maintain the upright position for at least 20 minutes after eating.

Appendix E

PROSODY

For the purposes of this work the following terms are used for non-verbal communication:

1. intonation, referring to variations in pitch;
2. stress, referring to degrees of loudness;
3. rate, referring to variations in speed of delivery;
4. pause, referring to periods of silence;
5. rhythm, referring to the movement and swing determined by thought and feeling;
6. timing, referring to the duration of different segments;
7. voice quality, referring to phonation;
8. resonance, referring to oral/nasal balance.

The comprehensive term for this whole area is 'prosody'.

Even in the most severe cases of some disorders of language and/or speech it is possible to determine the mother tongue of the language being attempted by the traces of intonation, stress and other recognizable non-verbal forms heard. Crystal (1969, 1973) points out that some of the prosodic characteristics of adult language are already discernible in the babbling of 6 to 7 month-old infants and that it is possible to trace utterances such as 'allgone' and 'ta' to the 8-month stage by means of the intonation and other prosodic features used.

Menyuk (1972), in her table of speech production and perception during the first year of life, claims the even earlier appearance of prosody. Her first allusion to prosody is as follows:

Stage II: at 3 weeks
Pseudo cry and non-cry utterances. There are a variety of temporal and frequency patterns.
Stage III: at 4 to 5 months
Babbling and the production of intoned utterances.
Utterances becoming increasingly more speech-like until the first year.
Stage IV; at 5 to 6 months
Increasing evidence of sensitivity to intonation and rhythm. Discrimination of intonational patterns and possibly segmental features (p. 15).

She goes on to state that some of the first aspects of speech the child observes both in production and in perception appear to be the supra-segmental aspects of the utterance, i.e. the prosodic and gestural aspects.

Cruttenden (1979) suggests that during the early months of life infants show a considerable command of the *forms* of intonation but nothing like an adult command of its *functions*. Several sources claim that a major part of assessment of an infant's later language/speech development can be predicted from careful informal listening to early productions and from the ability of the child to tune into the to-and-fro interaction with an adult at babble level. This is especially so when the adult uses the infant's intonations with expatiation, that is expanding the child's utterances and adding new information at the same time. Infant reaction to jingles, singing and music generally should also be noted.

Consideration of the appropriate unit of analysis employed by infants to decode 'heard' speech and to produce their own speech productions has been made by several workers. For example, Hawkins (1984) contrasts 'top-down' and 'bottom-up' approaches. She suggests that a child using a 'top-down' system would have a general schema for an over-all prosodic frame into which segments are gradually fitted. A child using a 'bottom-up' system would learn to integrate gestures for sub-syllabic and syllabic units, and in so doing arrive at an overall prosodic frame. Or possibly the child uses both systems simultaneously. Those studying child phonology originally thought that most children acquired phonology by the 'bottom-up' system. This did not take into account prosody or prosodic context (Waterson, 1970, 1971; Menn, 1978; Macken, 1979).

References

Albery, E.H. and Russell, J. (1990) Cleft palate and orofacial abnormalities in *Developmental Speech Disorders*, (ed. P. Grunwell), Churchill Livingstone, Edinburgh.

Albery, E.H., Hathorn, I.S. and Pigott, R.W. (1986) *Cleft Lip and Palate*, Wright, London.

Anthony, A., Bogle, D. and McIsaac, M.W. (1971) *The Edinburgh Articulation Test*, Livingstone, Edinburgh.

Andrews, G. and Harris, M. (1964) *The Syndrome of Stuttering*, Spastics Society Medical Education and Information Unit, London.

Andrews, G., Craig, A., Feyer, A.M., Hoddinott, S., Howie, P. and Neilson, M. (1983) Stuttering: a review of research findings and theories, *Journal of Speech and Hearing Disorders*, **48**, 226–46.

Andrews, S., Warner, J. and Stewart, R. (1986) EMG biofeedback and relaxation in the treatment of hyperfunctional dysphonia, *British Journal of Disorders of Communication*, **21**, no. 3, 353–69.

Aronson, A.E. (1985) *Clinical Voice Disorders*, 2nd edn, Thieme Inc., New York.

Ayres, A.J. (1972) *Southern California Sensory Integration Test*, Western Psychological Services, Los Angeles.

Basser, L.S. (1962) Hemiplegia of early onset and the faculty of speech with special reference to the effects of hemispherectomy, *Brain*, **85**, 427–60.

Bates, E. (1976) *Language and Context: the acquisition of pragmatics*, Academic Press, London.

BBC (1989) *Antennae*,

Beaumont, J.C. (1983) *Introduction to Neuropsychology*, Blackwell Scientific Publications, London.

Bernstein, D.A. and Borkovec, T.D. (1973) *Progressive Relaxation Training. A manual for the caring professions*, Research Press, Champaign, Illinois.

Beveridge, M. and Conti-Ramsden, G. (1987) *Children with Language Disabilities*, Open University Press, Milton Keynes.

Beveridge, M. and Lloyd, P. (1977) 'The developing person as a communicator', paper presented at the Annual Conference of the Developmental Section of the British Psychological Society, Cambridge.

Bicknell, J. (1983) *Bulletin of the Royal College of Psychiatrists*, **7**, 168.

Blakemore, C. (1988) The mind machine, *Horizon*, BBC 2.

Bloodstein, O.N. (1960a) Development of stuttering 1, *Journal of Speech and Hearing Disorders*, **25**, 219–37.

Bloodstein, O.N. (1960b) Development of stuttering 2, *Journal of Speech and Hearing Disorders*, **25**, 366–76.

Bloodstein, O.N. (1961) Development of stuttering 3, *Journal of Speech and Hearing Disorders*, **26**, 67–82.

Bloodstein, O.N. (1970) Stuttering and normal non-fluency – a continuity hypothesis, *British Journal of Disorders of Communication*, **5**, 30–9.

Bloom, L. and Lahey, M. (1978) *Language Development and Language Disorders*, Wiley and Sons, London.

Bloomfield, L. (1933) *Language*, Holt, Rinehart and Winstone, London.

Bluma, S., Shearer, M., Frohman, A. and Hilliard, J. (1976) *Manual of the Portage Guide to Early Education*, NFER, Windsor.

Bromley, D.B. (1974) *The Psychology of Human Ageing*, Penguin, Harmondsworth.

Brookshire, B.L., Lynch, J.I. and Fox, D.R. (1980) Feeding the infant and child with a cleft lip/palate, in *Child Cleft Palate Curriculum* (ed. B.L. Brookshire), C.C. Publications.

Brown, B.J. and Lloyd, H. (1975) A controlled study of children not speaking at school, *Journal of the Association of Workers for Maladjusted Children*, **3**, 49–63.

Bryant, M. (1980) Occupational Therapy, in *Helping Clumsy Children* (eds N. Gordon and I. McKinlay), Churchill Livingstone, London.

Byrne, R. (1983) *Let's Talk about Stammering*, Allen and Unwin, London.

Caplan, L. (1972) An investigation of some aspects of stuttering-like speech in adult dysphasic subjects, *Journal of the South African Speech and Hearing Association*, **19**, 52–66.

Chappell, G.E. (1973) Childhood verbal apraxia and its treatment, *Journal of Speech and Hearing Disorders*, **38** (3), 362–8.

Chappell, G.E. (1984) Developmental verbal dyspraxia: the expectant pattern, *Australian Journal of Human Communication Disorders*, **12** (2), 15–25.

Chomsky, N. (1957) *Syntactic Structures*, Mouton, The Hague.

Chumpelik, D. (1984) The Prompt System of Therapy: theoretical framework and applications for Developmental Apraxia of Speech, *Seminars in Speech and Language*, **5** (2), 139–54.

Code, C. (1987) *Language, Aphasia and the Right Hemisphere*, Wiley, London.

Cooper, M. (1973) *Modern Techniques of Vocal Rehabilitation*, C.C. Thomas, Springfield, Illinois.

Costello, J.M. (1983) Current behavioural treatments for children in *Treatment of Stuttering in Early Childhood* (eds D. Prins and R. Ingham), College Press, San Diego.

Cruttenden, A. (1979) *Language in Infancy and Childhood*, Manchester University Press, Manchester.

Crystal, D. (1969) *Prosodic Systems and Intonation in English*, Cambridge University Press, London.

Crystal, D. (1973) Linguistic mythology and the first year of life, *British Journal of Disorders of Communication*, **8** (1), 29–36.

Crystal, D. (1979) *Prosodic Development* in *Language Acquisition* (eds P. Fletcher and M. Garman), Cambridge University Press, Cambridge.

Crystal, D. (1981a) *Profiling Linguistic Disability*, Arnold, London.

Crystal, D. (1981b) *Clinical Linguistics*, Arnold, London.

Crystal, D., Fletcher, P. and Garman, M. (1976) *The Grammatical Analysis of Language Disability*, Arnold, London.

Culp, D.M. (1984) The preschool fluency development program: assessment and treatment in *Contemporary Approaches to Stuttering Therapy* (ed. M. Peins), Little, Brown and Co., Boston.

Cunningham, C. (1982) *Down's Syndrome: An introduction for parents*, Souvenir Press, London.

Cunningham, C., Cataldo, M.F., Mallion, C. and Keyes, J.B. (1983) A review and controlled single case evaluation of behavioural approaches to the management of elective mutism, *Child and Family Behaviour Therapy*, **5**, 87–94.

Cunningham, C., Glenn, S.M., Wilkinson, P. and Sloper, P. (1985) Mental ability, symbolic play and receptive and expressive language of young children with Down's syndrome, *Journal of Child Psychology and Psychiatry*, **26** (2), 255–65.

Dalton, P. and Hardcastle, W.J. (1977) *Disorders of Fluency and their Effects on Communication*, Arnold, London.

Daniloff, R.G., Hoffman, P., Alfonso, P. and Schuckers, G. (1981) 'Misarticulating children's perception of the VOT contrast', paper presented at the 102nd meeting of the Acoustical Society of America.

Darley, F.L., Aronson, A.E. and Brown, J.R. (1975) *Motor Speech Disorders*, W.B. Saunders Co., London.

David, R.D., Devel, R., Ferry, P. *et al.* (1981) 'Proposed nosology of disorders of higher cerebral function in children', Task Force on Nosology of Disorders of Higher Cerebral Function in Children, Child Neurology Society.

Dean, E. and Howell, J. (1986) Developing linguistic awareness: a theoretically based approach to phonological disorders, *British Journal of Disorders of Communication*, **21** (2), 223–38.

Denny-Brown, D. (1965) Physiological aspects of disturbances of speech, *Australian Journal of Experimental Biology and Medical Science*, **43**, 455–74.

DHSS (1972) Human Genetics, prepared by the Standing Medical Advisory Committee for the Central Health Services Council the Secretary of State for Social Services and the Secretary of State for Wales.

Diedrich, W.M. (1984) Cluttering: its diagnosis, in *Treating Articulation Disorders: for Clinicians by Clinicians* (ed. H. Winitz), University Park Press, Baltimore.

Dobbing, J. (1972) Growth of the Brain, in *The Human Brain*, Paladin, London (originally appeared as *Science Journal* Special Issue, May 1967).

DuBrul, E.L. (1958) *Evolution of the Speech Apparatus*, C. Thomas, Springfield, Illinois.

DuBrul, E.L. (1977) Origin of the speech apparatus and its reconstruction in fossils, *Brain and Language*, **4**, 365–81.

Dworkin, J.P. (1984) Specific characteristics and treatments of the dysarthrias, in *Treating Articulation Disorders: for Clinicians by Clinicians* (ed. H. Winitz), University Park Press, Baltimore.

Emery, O.B. (1986) Linguistic decrement in normal ageing, *Language and Communication*, **6** (1/2), 47–64.

Enderby, P. (1980) The Frenchay dysarthria assessment, *British Journal of Disorders of Communication*, **15** (3), 165–74.

Enderby, P. (1983) *The Frenchay dysarthria assessment*, College-Hill Press, San Diego.

Erikson, E.H. (1964) *Childhood and Society*, Penguin, London.

Fairbanks, G., Herbert, E. and Hammond, E. (1949) An acoustical study of vocal pitch in seven- and eight-year-old girls, *Child Development*, **20**, 71–4.

Ferguson, C.A. (1976) Learning to pronounce: the earliest stages of phonological development in the child, *Papers and Reports on Child Language Development*, **11**, 1–27.

Fransella, F. (1970) Stuttering: not a symptom but a way of life, *British Journal of Disorders of Communication*, **5**, 22–9.

Fransella, F. (1970) *Construct Theory, Psychotherapy and Stuttering*, Academic Press, London.

Fransella, F. (1972) *Personal Change and Reconstruction*, Academic Press, New York.

Fraser, G.M. and Blockley, J. (1973) *The Language Disordered Child*, NFER, London.

Froeschels, E. (1952) Chewing method as therapy, *Archives of Otolaryngology*, **56**, 427–34.

Frostig, M. and Horne, D. (1966) *Developmental Test of Visual Perception*, Consulting Psychologists' Press, Palo Alto.

Fry, D. (1977) *Homo Loquens: man as a talking animal*, Cambridge University Press, Cambridge.

Gaarder, K. and Chase, C. (1971) Control of states of consciousness, Part I: Attainment through external feedback augmenting control of psychophysiological variables, *Archives of General Psychiatry*, **25**, 429–35.

Gates, G.A. and Montalbo, P.J. (1987) The effects of low-dose Beta-blockade on performance anxiety in singers, *Journal of Voice*, **1** (1), 105–8.

Gerard, K. (1985) *Pre-linguistic Period of Language Development and the Development of Communicative Competence: Checklist*, Gerard, London.

Gornall, P., Jones, B. and Russell, V.J. (1983) 'Paediatric aspects of pre-surgical care', paper presented at 1st International meeting, Craniofacial Society of Great Britain, Birmingham.

Greene, M.C.L. (1980) *The Voice and its Disorders*, Pitman Press, Bath.

Greene, M.C.L. (1984) Functional dysphonia and the hyperventilation syndrome, *British Journal of Disorders of Communication*, **19** (3), 263–72.

Greene, M.G., Adelman, R., Charon, R. and Hoffman, S. (1986) Ageism in the medical encounter, *Language and Communication*, **6** (1/2), 113–24.

Grunwell, P. (1981) The development of phonology: a descriptive profile, *First Language*, **2**, 161–91.

Grunwell, P. (1985) *Phonological Assessment of Child Speech*, NFER-Nelson, Windsor.

Grunwell, P. and Russell, J. (1988) Phonological development in children with cleft lip and palate, *Clinical Linguistics and Phonetics*, **2** (2), 75–95.

Guyette, T.W. and Diedrich, W.M. (1981) A critical review of developmental apraxia of speech in *Speech and Language: Advances in basic research and practice, Vol. 5* (ed. N. J. Lass), Academic Press, New York.

Haberman, M. (1988) A mother of invention, *Nursing Times*, **84** (2) 52–3.

Hall, D. (1983) 'The role of the neuro-developmental examination in the assessment of children with special needs', paper presented at the Spastics Society Meeting on Screening Procedures in Child Health Clinics, Cambridge.

Halliday, M.A.K. (1975) *Learning How to Mean*, Edward Arnold, London.

Hardyck, C. and Petrinovitch, L.F. (1977) Left-handedness, *Psychological Bulletin*, **44**, 385–404.

Harri, M. and Tillemans, T. (1984) Conductive education, in *Management of the Motor Disorders of Children with Cerebral Palsy* (ed. D. Scrutton), Spastic International Medical Publications, London.

Harris, J. and Cottam, P. (1985) Phonetic features and phonological features in speech assessment, *British Journal of Disorders of Communication*, **20** (1), 61–74.

Hartley, X.Y. (1982) Receptive language processing of Down's syndrome children, *Journal of Mental Deficiency Research*, **26**, 263–9.

Hawkins, S. (1984) On the development of motor control in speech: evidence from studies of temporal co-ordination, in *Speech and Language: Advances in basic Research and Practice, Vol. 11*, Academic Press, New York.

Henderson, S.E. (1987) The assessment of 'clumsy' children: old and new approaches, *Journal of Child Psychology and Psychiatry*, **28** (4), 511–27.

Hogg, J. and Moss, S. (1983) 'The development of skilled motor sequences in Down's syndrome children', final report to Joseph Rowntree Memorial Fund.

Hollien, H. and Muller, E. (1973) Perceptual responses to infant crying: identification of cry types, *Journal of Child Language*, **1**, 89–95.

Howell, J. and Dean, E. (1987) 'I think that's a noisy sound': reflection and learning in the therapeutic situation, *Child Language, Teaching and Therapy*, **3** (3), 259–66.

Ineichen, B. (1984) Prevalence of mental illness among mentally handicapped people, *Journal of the Royal Society of Medicine*, **77**, 761–5.

Ingram, D. (1979) Phonological patterns in the speech of young children, in *Language Acquisition* (eds P. Fletcher and M. Garman), Cambridge University Press, Cambridge.

Jacobson, E. (1938) *Progressive Relaxation*, 2nd edn, The University of Chicago Press, Chicago.

Jaffe, M.B. (1984) Neurological impairment of speech production: assessment and treatment, in *Speech Disorders in Children* (ed. J. Costello), NFER-Nelson, Windsor.

Jesperson, O. (1922) *Language: its nature, development and origin*, Allen and Unwin, London.

Johnson, W. (1959) *The Onset of Stuttering: Research findings and implications*. University of Minneapolis Press, Minneapolis.

Jones, O. (1975) 'A comparative study of early mother-child communication, with young normal children and young Down's syndrome children', paper presented at the Loch Lomond symposium on communicative development, University of Strathclyde, Glasgow.

Kelly, G.A. (1955) *The Psychology of Personal Constructs*, **2**, I and II. Norton, New York.

Kempson R. (1977) *Semantic Theory*, Cambridge University Press, Cambridge.

Kent, R.D. (1976) Anatomical and neuromuscular maturation of the speech mechanism. Evidence from acoustic studies, *Journal of Speech and Hearing Research*, **19**, 422–47.

Kent, R.D. (1981) Articulatory-acoustic perspectives on speech development, in *Language Behaviour in Infancy and Childhood* (ed. R.E. Stark), Elsevier-North Holland, Amsterdam.

Kent, R.D. (1982) Sensorimotor aspects of speech development, in *Development of perception: psychobiological perspectives* (eds R.N. Aslin, J.R. Alberts and M.R. Peterson), Academic, vol. 1, New York.

Kent, R.D. (1984) Psychobiology of speech development: co-emergence of language and a movement system, *American Journal of Physiology*, **246** (6), R889-R894.

Kent, R.D. (1985) Stuttering as a temporal programming disorder, in *Nature and Treatment of Stuttering. New directions* (eds R.F. Curlee and W.H. Perkins), Taylor and Francis, London.

Kent, R.D. and Netsell, R. (1975) A case study of an ataxic dysarthric: cineradiographic and spectrographic observations, *Journal of Speech and Hearing Disorders*, **40**, 115–34.

Kertesz, A. and Hooper, P. (1982) Praxis and language: the extent and variety of apraxia in aphasia, *Neuropsychologia*, **20**, 275–86.

Klick, S.L. (1985) Adapted cuing technique for use in the treatment of dyspraxia, *Language, Speech and Hearing Services in Schools*, **6** (4), 256–60.

Kolb, B. and Milner, B. (1979) cited in B. Kolb and I.Q. Wishaw (eds) (1979) *Fundamentals of Human Neuropsychology*, W.H. Freeman, San Francisco.

Kools, J.A. and Tweedie, D. (1975) Development of praxis in children, *Perceptual and Motor Skills*, **40**, 11–19.

Kolvin, J. and Fundudis, T. (1981) Elective mute children. Psychological development and background factors, *Journal of Child Psychology and Psychiatry*, **22**, 219–33.

Kugler, P.N., Kelso, J.A.S. and Turvey, M.T. (1980) On the concept of co-ordinative structures, I. Theoretical lines of convergence, in *Tutorials in Motor Behaviour* (eds G.E. Stelmach and J. Requin), Elsevier-North Holland, Amsterdam.

Laitman, J.T. and Crelin, P. (1976) Postnatal development of the basicranium and the vocal tract region in man, in *Symposium on Development of the Basicranium* (ed. J.F. Bosma), DHEW Publications, NIH 76–989.

Langley, J. (1988) *Working with Swallowing Disorders*, Winslow Press, Bicester.

Lee, V. (ed.) (1979) *Language Development*, Croom Helm, London.

Lenneberg, E.H. (1967) *Biological Foundations of Language*, John Wiley and Sons Inc., New York.

Le Prevost, P.A. (1983) Using the Makaton vocabulary in early language training with a Down's baby: a single case study, *Mental Handicap*, **11**, 28.

Lerman, J.W. (1980) Disorders of phonation and their management, *Ear, Nose and Throat Journal*, **59**, 62–73.

Lewis, M. (1936) *Infant Speech: a study of the beginning of language*, Harcourt Brace, New York.

Lorenz, K.Z. (1961) *King Solomon's Ring*, Methuen, London.

Luchsinger, R. and Arnold, G.E. (1965) *Voice-Speech-Language*, Wadsworth Pub. Co. Inc., Belmont, California.

Luria, A.R. (1966) *Higher Cortical Functions in Man*, Basic Books, New York.

Luria, A.R. (1973) *The Working Brain*, Penguin, London.

Luria, A.R. and Yudovich F. la (1971) *Speech and the Development of Mental Processes in the Child*, Penguin Education, London.

Lynch, J.I., Fox, D.R. and Brookshire, B.L. (1983) Phonological proficiency of two cleft palate toddlers with school age follow-up, *Journal of Speech and Hearing Disorders*, **48**, 274–85.

McClean, N. (1977) Effects of auditory masking on lip movements during speech, *Journal of Speech and Hearing Research*, **20**, 731–41.

Macken, M.A. (1979) Developmental reorganisation in phonology, *Lingua*, **49**, 11–49.

Martin, J.A.M. (1981) *Voice, Speech and Language in the Child*, Springer-Verlag Wien, New York.

Martin, S. (1988) Are your patients running in vocal marathons? *Speech Therapy in Practice*, **4** (3), 5.

McGlone, R.E. (1978) Sex differences in functional brain asymmetry, *Cortex*, **14**, 122–8.

McGlone, R.E. (1983) Sex differences in human brain organisation: a critical survey, *The Behavioural and Brain Sciences*, **3**, 215–27.

McGlone, R.E. and Brown, W. (1969) Identification of 'shift' between vocal registers, *Journal of the Acoustical Society of America*, **46**, 1033–6.

McGlone, R.E. and McGlone, H. (1972) Speaking fundamental frequency of 8 year-old girls, *Folia Phoniatrica*, **24**, 313–17.

Menn, L. (1978) Phonological units in beginning speech in *Syllables and Segments* (eds A. Bell and J.P. Hooper), Elsevier-N. Holland, Amsterdam.

Menn, L. (1980) Phonological theory and child phonology, in *Child Phonology, Vol. I, Production* (eds G.H. Yeni-Komshian, J.F. Kavanagh and C.A. Ferguson), Academic Press, London.

Menyuk, P. (1972) *The Development of Speech*, Bobbs Merrill Co., New York.

Miller, G.A. (1951) *Language and Communication*, McGraw-Hill Inc., New York.

Milloy, N.R. (1985) 'The assessment and identification of developmental articulatory dyspraxia and its effect on phonological development', unpublished Ph.D. thesis, Leicester Polytechnic.

Milloy, N.R. (1988) *What is Dyspraxia?* Vocal, London.

Milloy, N.R. and Morgan-Barry, R. (1990) Developmental neurological disorders, in *Developmental speech disorders* (ed. P. Grunwell), Churchill Livingstone, Edinburgh.

Milloy, N.R. and Summers, L. (1989) Six years on – do claims still hold?: four children reassessed on a procedure to identify developmental articulatory dyspraxia, *Child Language, Teaching and Therapy*, **5** (3), 287–303.

Moncur, J.P. and Brackett, I.P. (1974) *Modifying Vocal Behaviour*, Harper and Row, New York.

Moore, W.H. and Haynes, W.O. (1980) Alpha hemispheric asymmetry and stuttering: some support for a segmentation dysfunction hypothesis, *Journal of Speech and Hearing Research*, **23**, 229–97.

Morley, M.E. (1972) *The Development and Disorders of Speech in Childhood*, 3rd edn, Churchill Livingstone, Edinburgh.

Morris, R.J. and Brown, W.S. (1987) Age-related voice measures among adult women, *Journal of Voice*, **1** (1), 38–43.

Morrish, E.C.E. (1988) Compensatory articulation in a subject with total glossectomy, *British Journal of Disorders of Communication*, **23** (1), 13–22.

Moscovitch, M. (1981) Right hemisphere language. Adult language, *Topics in Language Disorders*, **1** (4), 41–62.

Nation, J.E. and Aram, D.M. (1977) *Diagnosis of Speech and Language Disorders*, Henry Kimpton, London.

Netsell, R. (1981) The acquisition of motor speech control: a perspective with directions for research, in *Language Behaviour in Infancy and Early Childhood* (ed. R.E. Stark), Elsevier-North Holland, Oxford.

Netsell, R. (1986) *A Neurobiologic View of Speech Production and the Dysarthrias*, Taylor and Francis, London.

Penfield, W. and Rasmussen, T. (1950) *The Cerebral Cortex of Man: a clinical study of localisation of function*, Macmillan, New York.

Perkins, W.H. (1977) *Speech Pathology: an applied behavioural science*, 2nd edn. Mosby, St Louis.

Perry, A. (1988) Surgical voice restoration following laryngectomy: the tracheo-oesophageal fistula technique (Singer-Blom), *British Journal of Disorders of Communication*, **23** (1), 23–30.

Perry, A. and Edels, Y. (1985) Recent advances in the assessment of failed oesopageal speakers, *British Journal of Disorders of Communication*, **20** (3), 229–38.

Peters, H.F.M. (1986) 'Limitations and possibilities in speech motor behaviour in stuttering', presented at the International Symposium on Physiology and Therapy in Stuttering, Brussels.

Peto, A. (1955) Konductiv mozgasterapia mint gyogypedagogia, *Gyogypedagogia*, **1**, 15–21.

Piaget, J. (1956) *The Child's Conception of Space*, Routledge and Kegan Paul, London.

Prutting, C.A. (1982) Pragmatics as social competence, *Journal of Speech and Hearing Disorders*, **47** (2), 123–34.

Quin, V. and Macauslan, A. (1986) *Dyslexia*, Penguin, London.

Ramig, L.A. (1986) Aging speech, *Language and Communication*, **6** (1/2), 25–34.

Ramig, L.A. and Ringel, R. (1983) Effect of physiological ageing on select characteristics of voice, *Journal of Speech and Hearing Research*, **26**, 22–50.

Rapin, I. (1982) *Children with Brain Dysfunction*, Raven Press, New York.

Rasmussen, T. and Milner, B. (1977) The role of early left brain injury in determining lateralisation of cerebral speech functions, *Annals of New York Academy of Sciences*, **299**, 355–69.

Reed, G.F. (1963) Elective mutism in children: a reappraisal, *Journal of Child Psychology and Psychiatry*, **4**, 99–107.

Richards, M. (1980) *Infancy: World of the newborn*, Harper and Row, London.

Riley, D.R. and Riley, J. (1984) A component model for treating stuttering in children, in *Contemporary Approaches to Stuttering Therapy* (ed. M. Peins), Little, Brown and Co., Boston.

Ritchie Russell, W. and Dewar, A.J. (1975) *Explaining the Brain*, Oxford University Press, Oxford.

Roach, E.G. and Kephart, N.C. (1966) *The Purdue Perceptual-Motor Survey*, Charles D. Merrill, Columbus, Ohio.

Roach, P.J. and Hardcastle, W.J. (1974) *A Computer System for the Processing of Electropalatographic and Other Articulatory Data*, Phonetics Laboratory, Department of Linguistic Science, University of Reading.

Robertson, S.J. (1982) *Dysarthria Profile*, Robertson, London.

Rondal, J.A. (1978) Maternal speech to normal children and Down's syndrome children matched for mean length of utterances, in *Behaviour in the Profoundly and Severely Retarded: Research foundations for enhancing the quality of life* (ed. C.E. Myers), American Association on Mental Deficiency, Washington, D.C.

Rosenbek, J. (1980) Apraxia of speech – relationship to stuttering, *Journal of Fluency Disorders*, **5**, 233–53.

Russell, J. (1989) Early intervention in *Cleft Palate: Nature and remediation of communicative problems* (ed. J. Stengelhofen), Churchill Livingstone, Edinburgh.

Rustin, L. (1987) *Assessment and Therapy Programme for Dysfluent Children*, NFER-Nelson, London.

Rustin, L., Ryan, B.P. and Ryan, B.V. (1987) Use of the Monterey programmed stuttering therapy in Great Britain, *British Journal of Disorders of Communication*, **22** (2), 151–62.

Ryan, B. (1974) *Programmed Therapy for Stuttering Children and Adults*, Thomas, Springfield, Illinois.

Ryan, W.J. and Burk, K.W. (1974) Perceptual and acoustic correlates of ageing in the speech of males, *Journal of Communication Disorders*, **7**, 181–92.

Sand, P.L. and Taylor, N. (1973) Handedness: evaluation of the binomial distribution hypothesis in children and adults, *Perceptual and Motor Skills*, **36**, 1343–6.

Sapir, S. and Aronson, A.E. (1985) Aphonia after closed head injury: aetiologic considerations, *British Journal of Disorders of Communication*, **20**, 286–96.

Schmidt, R.A. (1975a) *Motor Skills*, Harper and Row, New York.

Schmidt, R.A. (1975b) A schema theory of discrete motor skill learning, *Psychological Review*, **82**, 225–60.

Schmidt, R.A. (1976) The schema as a solution to some persistent problems in motor learning theory, in *Motor Control: Issues and trends* (ed. G. Stelmach), Academic Press, New York.

Scholefield, J.A. (1987) Aetiologies of aphonia following closed head injury, *British Journal of Disorders of Communication*, **22** 167–72.

Schultz, J.A. and Luthe, W. (1959) *Autogenic Training*, Grune and Stratton, New York.

Segalowitz, S.T. and Bryden, M.P. (1983) Individual differences in hemispheric representations of language, in *Language Functions and Brain Organisation* (ed. S.J. Segalowitz), Academic Press, London.

Selley, W.G. and Boxall, J. (1986) A new way to treat sucking and swallowing difficulties in babies, *The Lancet*, **8491**, 1182–4.

Sharkey, S.G. and Folkins, J.W. (1985) Variability of lip and jaw movements in children and adults: implications for the development of motor speech control, *Journal of Speech and Hearing Research*, **28**, 8–15.

Sheehan, J.G. (1975) Conflict theory and avoidance-reduction therapy in *Stuttering: a second symposium* (ed. J. Eisenson), Harper and Rowe, New York.

Sheehan, J.G. and Martyn, M.M. (1970) Stuttering and its disappearance, *Journal of Speech and Hearing Research*, **13**, 279–89.

Shine, R. (1984) Assessment and fluency training with the young stutterer, in *Contemporary Approaches to Stuttering Therapy* (ed. M. Peins), Little, Brown and Co., Boston.

Simpson, J.A. (1954) Aphonia and deafness in hyperparathyroidism, *British Medical Journal*, **4869**, 494.

Singer, M.I. and Blom, E.D. (1980) An endoscopic technique for restoration of voice after laryngectomy, *Annals of Otology, Rhinology and Laryngology*, **89**, 529–33.

Sluckin, A. (1977) Children who do not talk at school, *Child: Care, health and development*, **3**, 69–79.

Sluckin, A., Foremans, N. and Herbert, M. (1990) Selective mutism: factors influencing selectivity of speaking at follow-up, *Australian Psychologist*, Australian Psychological Society, Parkevale, Melbourne.

Smith, A. and Luschei, E. (1983) Assessment of oral-motor reflexes in stutterers and normal speakers: preliminary observations, *Journal of Speech and Hearing Research*, **26**, 322–8.

Smith, R. (1988) Pragmatics and speech pathology in *Theoretical Linguistics and Disordered Language*, (ed. M. Ball), Croom Helm, London.

Sorenson, D.N. (1989) Fundamental frequency investigation of children aged 6;0 to 10;0, *Journal of Communication Disorders*, **22**, 115–23.

Southall, D.P., Stebbens, V.A., Mirza, R. *et al.* (1987) Upper airway obstruction with hypoxaemia and sleep disruption in Down's syndrome, *Developmental Medicine and Child Neurology*, **29** (6), 734–42.

Sparks, R.W. and Holland, A.L. (1976) Method: melodic intonation therapy for aphasia, *Journal of Speech and Language Disorders*, **41**, 287–97.

Spirduso, W.W. (1982) Physical fitness in relation to motor aging in *The Aging Motor System* (eds J.A. Mortimer, F.J. Pirrozzolo and G.J. Maletta), Praeger, New York.

St. James-Roberts, I. (1981) A re-interpretation of hemispherectomy data without functional plasticity of brain, *Brain and Language*, **13**, 31–53.

Stark, R.E., Rose, S.N. and McLagen, M. (1975) Features of infant sounds: the first 8 weeks of life, *Journal of Child Language*, **2**, 205–31.

Stark, R.E. (1980) Stages of speech development in the first year of life, in *Child Phonology, Vol. I, Production* (eds G.H. Yeni-Komshian, J.F. Kavanagh and C.A. Ferguson) Academic Press, New York.

Steig Pearce, P., Darwish, H.Z. and Gaines, B.H. (1987) Visual symbol and manual sign learning by children with phonological programming deficit syndrome, *Developmental Medicine and Child Neurology*, **29**, 743–50.

Stemple, J. (1984) *Clinical Voice Pathology: Theory and management*, Merrill Pub. Co., Columbus, Ohio.

Stemple, J. and Bailey, J. (1982) 'The Lombard reflex as a test of vocal hyperfunction in children', paper presented at A-S-L-H-A Convention, Toronto.

Stemple, J. and Lehmann, D. (1980) 'Throat clearing: the unconscious habit of vocal hyperfunction', paper presented at A-S-L-H-A Convention, Detroit.

Stern, D.N., Jaffe, J., Beebe, B. and Bennet, S.L. (1975) Vocalising in unison and in alternation: two modes of communication within the mother-infant dyad, *Annals of New York Academy of Sciences*, **263**, 89–100.

Stoel-Gammon, C. (1980) Phonological analysis of four Down's syndrome children, *Applied Psycholinguistics*, **1**, 31–48.

Stott, D.H., Moyes, F.A. and Henderson, S.E. (1984) *The Henderson Revision of the Test of Motor Impairment*, Psychological Corporation, San Antonio.

Straight, H.S. (1980) Auditory versus articulatory phonological processes and their development in children, in *Child Phonology, Vol. I, Production* (eds G.H. Yeni-Komshian, J.F. Kavanagh and C.A. Ferguson), Academic Press, New York.

Sylvester, P.E. (1983) Aging in the mentally retarded, in *First European Symposium Issue*, Royal Society of Medicine, London.

Talbot, L. (1988) Feeding problems in at-risk infants need consistent management, *Speech Therapy in Practice*, **4** (1), 22–4.

Thelen, E. (1981) Rhythmical behaviour in infancy: an ethological perspective, *Developmental Psychology*, **17**, 237–57.

Thibodeau, L.M. and Sussman, H.M. (1979) Performance on a test of categorical perception of speech in normal and communicatively disordered children, *Journal of Phonetics*, **7**, 375–91.

Tough, J. (1977) *The Development of Meaning*, Unwin Educational, London.

Treharne, D.A. (1980) Feeding patterns and speech development in *Language Disability in Children* (ed. F.M. Jones), MTP Press, Lancaster.

Trost, J.E. (1971) 'Apraxia dysfluency in patients with Broca's aphasia', paper presented at the annual convention of ASHA, Chicago.

Van Riper, C. (1971) *The Nature of Stuttering*, Prentice Hall, Engelwood Cliffs, New Jersey.

Van Riper, C. (1973) *The Treatment of Stuttering*, Prentice Hall, Englewood Cliffs, New Jersey.

Ward, P.H., Engel, E. and Nance, W.E. (1968) The larynx in the Cri du Chat syndrome, *American Academy of Ophthalmology and Otolaryngology*, **72**, 90–102.

Wardough, R. (1985) *How Conversation Works*, Blackwell, Oxford.

Warner, J. (1981) *Helping the Handicapped Child with Early Feeding. A checklist and manual for parents and professionals*, PTM, Winslow.

Warnock, M. (1979) Children with special educational needs: the Warnock Report, *British Medical Journal*, **1**, 667–8.

Wasz-Hockert, O., Lind, J., Vuorenkoski, V. *et al.* (1968) *The Infant Cry*, Heinemann Medical Books, London.

Waterson, N. (1970) 'Some speech forms of an English child: a phonological study', transactions of the Philological Society, London.

Waterson, N. (1971) Child phonology. A prosodic view. *Journal of Linguistics*, **7**, 179–211.

Weiss, D.A. (1964) *Cluttering*, Prentice Hall Inc., Engelwood Cliffs, New Jersey.

Weistuch, L. and Byers Brown, B. (1987) Motherese as therapy: a programme and its dissemination, *Child Language, Teaching and Therapy*, **3** (1), 57–71.

Wingate, M.E. (1967) Stuttering and word length, *Journal of Speech and Hearing Research*, **10**, 146–52.

Wingate, M.E. (1976) *Stuttering: Theory and treatment*, Irvington, New York.

Wischner, G.J. (1969) Stuttering behaviour, learning theory and behaviour therapy; problems, issues and progress in *Stuttering and the Conditioning Therapies* (eds B.B. Gray and G. England), Monterey Institute for Speech and Hearing, Monterey, California.

Wolff, P. (1979) 'Theoretical issues in the development of motor skills'. Symposium on developmental disabilities in the pre-school child, Johnson and Johnson, Chicago.

Wolk, L. (1986) Cluttering: a diagnostic case report, *British Journal of Disorders of Communication*, **21** (2), 199–208.

Worster-Drought, C. (1974) *Suprabulbar Paresis*, Supplement to Developmental Medicine and Child Neurology, Heinemann Medical Publications, London.

Author Index

Subject index